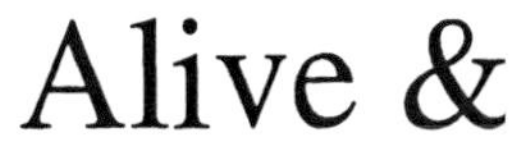

Alive &

Volume Two

Into The New Millennium With Edgar Cayce's Health Care Wisdom

by Bette S. Margolis

Published by
Transpersonal
Publishing
www.TranspersonalPublishing.com

Alive & Well: Volume Two
Into The New Millennium With Edgar Cayce's Health Care Wisdom (Revised Edition)

Edgar Cayce Readings
Edgar Cayce Foundation

This Title- Volume Two; ISBN 1-929661-13-4
First Printing, April, 2003
Second Printing, Revised, January, 2005

Volume One: ISBN 1-929661-12-6

For additional copies, retail, or wholesale quantities of this book or other related books, tapes, and CDs, contact the publisher through the worldwide web:

www.TranspersonalPublishing.com

Transpersonal Publishing
A Division of AHU, LLC
PO Box 249
Goshen, VA 24439

Manufactured in the United States of America
10 9 8 7 6 5 4 3 2 1

....

FOREWORD

David McMillin, MA,
Researcher, Meridian Institute

As a researcher of the Edgar Cayce health information, I have developed a great appreciation for the historical and conceptual context of Cayce's life and work. Edgar Cayce was a medical intuitive who gave psychic "readings" for persons suffering from a broad range of conditions. The content of his health readings were clearly linked to the medical and personal resources that were available during his era (early twentieth century).

These resources changed over the years and the Cayce readings adapted to the new context. The period of Cayce's life was rich with new and exciting therapeutic techniques and systems of healing, much as it is today with complementary and alternative medicine, integrative medicine, functional medicine, etc. The diverse range of therapeutic options available to Cayce is clearly evident in the treatment plans that he prescribed. With new products and services continuously becoming available and others fading just as quickly, Cayce's intuitive process was flexible and adaptive in choosing the optimal remedies for an individual at any given point in time.

For example, for almost ten years Cayce recommended suspending a bottle of tincture of iodine into a simple chemical battery called a wet cell. The battery would be plugged into an electrical outlet and "charged" to enhance the effectiveness of the iodine. The iodine would then be used as part of an integrated treatment plan for that individual.

In 1931, Dr. Sunkar Bisey obtained a reading from Cayce on his iodine-based product Atomidine. The main ingredient in Dr. Bisey's Atomidine was iodine trichloride. In the trance state, Cayce endorsed the product but told

Dr. Bisey that it could be improved by charging it in a wet cell battery. Apparently Cayce must have been satisfied with Bisey's manufacturing process because almost from that time on, Cayce stopped giving readings on how to charge tincture of iodine in a wet cell battery. Instead, he simply prescribed Atomidine.

Atomidine became difficult to obtain in 1944, probably due to the death of Dr. Bisey and difficulty obtaining some of the ingredients for Atomidine. Keep in mind that the second world war was raging. In typical fashion, Cayce adapted to the situation by going back to recommending that tincture of iodine be charged in a wet cell battery, much as he had done in the years prior to 1931. Yet, the readings for charging iodine in 1944 were different than the earlier ones because by then, battery chargers were fairly common so the whole process was much easier and safer. Thus, Cayce adapted the process to fit the resources. Some modern producers of Atomidine-type products charge the iodine in a wet cell battery, just as Cayce recommended for Dr. Bisey. I have found many such stories in the Cayce health material.

Cayce's penchant for adaptation was not random. Although the therapeutic modalities that he recommended changed, the underlying principles of health and healing did not. Cayce insisted that the body has the innate ability to heal itself. This intrinsic ability is divine and manifests via a low form of electricity (as in the wet cell battery). The divine healing energy is spiritual, because we are, in essence, spiritual beings. Natural remedies that work with inborn healing forces are usually preferable, although any treatment can be utilized for good. Cayce often reminded us that, ***"Mind is the builder"***. (349-4) (11). Working with attitudes and emotions is an important aspect of healing. These are some of the principles that provided continuity to the Cayce readings over the decades.

Although therapies and the words we use to describe the therapeutic processes have changed, many of the underlying principles that Cayce endorsed are very much "alive and well". They are being applied today, as exemplified in the following chapters of this book. I found *Alive and Well* to be informative, easy-reading, written in a personal tone derived from the author's own journey. The chapters are like a buffet with assorted tasty selections containing a diversity that matches Cayce's scope. I believe you will, as I did, find *Alive and Well* stimulating and enjoyable reading.

David McMillin, MA,
Researcher, Meridian Institute
Virginia Beach, Virginia

CONTENTS

1

THE HEALING TOUCH

Janet Mentgen, RN, BSN, CHTP, CHTI,
Developer of Healing Touch

....

As the body attunes self...
it may be a channel where
there may even be instant healing
with the laying on of hands...

EDGAR CAYCE
Reading 281- 5

Healing Touch is the art of
caring that comes from the heart
of the healer and reaches to the
person who is receiving help.

Janet Mentgen, RN, BSN, CHTP, CHTI,
Developer of Healing Touch

The Healing Touch program is a multi-level educational program teaching many energy based therapies. Healing Touch was originated by Janet Mentgen and further developed by the American Holistic Nurses Association in 1990. Mentgen earned her BS in Nursing from the University of Colorado. She has over 25 years of nursing experience in energy-based therapies, and is an international speaker and instructor of the Healing Touch. Mentgen is co-author of *Healing Touch Notebook I & II* and *Healing Touch: A Resource for Health Care Professionals.* She is a member of the American Nurses Association, Colorado Nurses Association, Canadian Holistic Nurses Association, Australia Holistic Nurses Association and Non-Practicing and Part-Time Nurses Association.

•••••••••••••••

...Healers offer purity of intention
and loving service. May the Divine
Spirit guide and ground those who
give and receive Healing Touch.

Janet Mentgen, RN, BSN, CHTP, CHTI,
Developer of Healing Touch

•••••••••••••••

INTERVIEW WITH JANET MENTGEN,
Developer of the Healing Touch

One of the oldest forms of health care known to man is healing with human energy. At the Colorado Center For Healing Touch, Lakewood, Colorado, experienced healers teach apprentices energy-based therapies that aid clientele in the process of self-healing. I was at their main offices for the following interview with Janet Mentgen, the Healing Touch program originator.

BETTE: What is the Healing Touch, Janet?

JANET: Healing Touch is a way of caring and a way of touching that relaxes the client. Relaxation shifts the client's energy field influencing the self-healing process. All healing is self-healing that comes from an individual, not the healer. To self-heal one needs to surrender to the spiritual source in the deepest core within our being. The process can be activated cooperatively between therapist and client. The healer's energy is systematically used to improve the client's energetic field. During a Healing Touch session the healer often experiences health changes too. I think of Healing Touch as an umbrella of the work of many healers who use energy-based techniques.

BETTE: What are these techniques used in Healing Touch?

JANET: There are dozens of them. The Hopi Indian Technique, for example, is used for functional back problems. It clears energy blockages and repairs vertebrae. Another maneuver is the Scudder Technique, developed by Rev. John Scudder of Illinois. This is a light touch method that induces relaxation by brushing accumulated energy down the major meridians and away from the joints. A Healing Touch approach that I developed is the Magnetic Unruffle, a long continuous raking motion. The hands move in the energy field above the body of the client who is lying down on his/her back. It begins with the healer's hands approximately 12 inches above the client's head. Then the healer's hands move approximately 2 inches away from the body, down to the center of the body, to the feet and then off the body.

The names of several other Healing Touch therapies are: Vertebral Spiral Technique, Spiral Meditation Technique, Mind Clearing and Pain Drain. Another one is Chakra Spread, a technique producing a deep healing that opens the major chakras throughout the body. In the readings, Edgar Cayce identifies the gonads, cells of Leydig, adrenals, thymus, thyroid, pineal and the pituitary as the 7 glands or chakras that transmit vortexes of energy. Chakra is a Sanskrit word meaning spinning wheel. It is the chakras that play an especially important role as the 7 major spiritual centers of our body connecting us with the Divine. Dr. Brugh Joy, MD, developed the Chakra Connection, a method created to balance the body's energy by directing energy from chakra to chakra. This maneuver facilitates a connection between all major energy centers in the body.

BETTE: How many chakras, major and minor, are in the human body?

JANET: There are 49 minor and 7 major chakras, according to Alice Bailey author of *Esoteric Healing*. The minor chakras are located in the hands, elbows, knees, ankles, feet, hips, spleen, fingers and toes. The major chakras are called: Root, Sacral, Solar Plexus, Heart, Throat, Brown and Crown. In the Edgar Cayce readings, Cayce refers to the Eastern chakras, but changes their order slightly. He links the chakras with the 7 main endocrine glands as major spiritual centers in the human body that play an important role in connection with the Divine.

BETTE: What do chakras look like?

JANET: Chakras are spinning, cone-shaped vortices of energy connected through a line paralleling the spinal column. Chakras are wide at the opening on the outside of the body and narrow at the base extending out of the front and back of the body. The crown chakra, located at the top of the head, extends upward, and it extends downward at its base. Each chakra has a specific location, purpose, special focus, color, psychological functions, an emotion, a gland that it affects and an area of the body that it governs. For example, the purpose of the crown chakra is the spiritual aspect. The focus of the crown chakra is on higher will. Its color is violet-white. Understanding, oneness, and knowing is the crown chakra's psychological functioning. Its emotion is bliss, and the pineal gland is the area of the body that the crown chakra affects. Chakras are like master switches that move and distribute energy throughout the body. They interface with the physical body through the endocrine glands.

BETTE: Would you classify Healing Touch as a religious program?

JANET: Healing Touch falls into the spiritual category. We believe that religion is an individual's choice. Our program is open to any religious belief. Healing Touch practitioners are encouraged to use their religious background for the highest good in their work as healers.

BETTE: How do you define spirituality?

JANET: For me spirituality is the holism of one true God. It is emulated in a balance of physical, emotional, mental and spiritual health. We have many books available to our students on spirituality, spiritual healing, meditation and the Laying On Of Hands. Healing Touch Spiritual Ministry is one of our programs that uses these books. The program is available to parish and hospice nurses, prayer teams, clergy and religious groups. The Laying On Of Hands and other energy-based healing techniques are taught from a Judaeo-Christian perspective. We offer certification programs primarily to people in healing professions. Healing Touch works well as a complement to nursing, conventional and alternative medicine, chiropractic, psychotherapy, counseling, physical therapy, massage, reiki and polarity therapy.

BETTE: Can lay people learn Healing Touch?

JANET: Yes, a lay person can learn Healing Touch to use on family members, for first aid intervention or for personal use. My children and grandchildren do Healing Touch. They were raised with it and think it is a normal way of life.

BETTE: What scientific studies have confirmed that human touch can initiate self-healing?

JANET: One of the first studies was conducted in 1961 by Canadian biologist Bernard Grad. He placed 300 wounded mice into 3 experimental groups: Group one was allowed to heal without intervention; group two was cared for by medical students; and group three was held by Oskar Estebany, a known healer. Accelerated wound healing was evident in the group of mice held by Estebany. Scientific studies done since 1986 on the human energy system maintain the use of Healing Touch in accelerated wound healing, relief of pain, increased relaxation, reduction of anxiety and stress, prevention of illness, energizing the field, enhancement of spiritual development, easing the dying process and as support in preparation for and after medical treatments and procedures.

BETTE: What is the human energy system?

JANET: Various cultures have given human energy or life essence different names: Chi, Qi, Prana, Life Force, Ki, Orgone, Life Energy and Universal Force. The human energy system is a biofield of electromagnetic energy surrounding and flowing through the body. It is beyond the normal range of ordinary detection, but can be identified with the hands. There are 3 parts to the human energy system: The energy field or aura is part one. Some people can clairvoyantly perceive the human aura or energy field surrounding the body like an envelope. The energy centers or chakras are part two. And the energy tracts known as meridians or pathways that facilitate energy throughout the body are part three. The three parts of the human energy system function independently and influence all aspects of an individual's life. Every experience, thought, memory or feeling is reflected in the human aura. Distortions in the energy system affect our physical and emotional health, mental patterns and spiritual awareness before becoming an actual symptom. Apprentices of the Healing Touch are given instructions by trained healers on determining, balancing, repairing, repatterning and aligning a distorted energy system. They are also taught how to recharge depleted areas of energy and how to clear blocked energy in the human energy field.

BETTE: What does the aura look like?

JANET: When the aura is healthy it is a clear, vibrant, fluid, fluffy substance with straight lines of force that facilitate energy exchange. There are 4 major layers to the auric field: etheric, emotional, mental and spiritual. According to former NASA physicist Barbara Brennan, the etheric field is the duplication of the physical body. Its structural field is 0.25 to 2 inches, and consists of light blue to gray lines of force. The etheric field can be seen with the peripheral vision. It resembles clouds, has rainbow colors, maintains continual fluid motion and extends 1 to 3 inches beyond the physical body. Emotions occur in the emotional field. The mental field, where mental ideas or thoughts are represented, is bright yellow. It resembles fine structural lines that stretch 3 to 8 inches from the body. There are 4 or more layers that assist us in connecting to our spirit. The spiritual field extends approximately 24 inches or more away from the body. People who are highly evolved spiritually can have an aura extending much further.

BETTE: Are there scientific observations of the human energy field?

JANET: Yes. A Japanese researcher named Montoyama did electronic measurements in 1984 confirming the existence of human energy fields with his calculations of the acupuncture meridians associated with the body's 7 major chakra areas along the outline of the spinal column. Also Kirlian photography, a unique photographic method, records on sensitive film the energy field surrounding all living things. Kirlian photography was also used by a group of physicians at a Madras, India hospital to photograph luminous auras of over 1000 patients. Brain tumor patients had flat auras on Kirlian photographs. Men with cirrhosis had branch-like auras. Individuals suffering with gastroenteritis had auras with streaks running parallel to the fingertips. Schizophrenics had misshapen auras. Researchers have also found Kirlian photography to be helpful in detecting cancer.

BETTE: What is the most interesting experience you have had administering Healing Touch?

JANET: I have had many interesting and rewarding experiences with various clients. One lady healed a fracture in 48 hours. It was the fastest bone healing I have ever seen. And she experienced minimal discomfort. The only thing that I did was an Unruffling and Ultrasound intervention on her within a minute or two after the accident. I put her in the shower to wash the gravel out of her arm and worked on her about 6 minutes as she stood under the running water. She went to her doctor who told her that her arm was broken. They x-rayed her 2 days later and her arm was healed.

BETTE: Do you possess special healing powers?

JANET: I don't think I am a miraculous person. I believe I was able to relax this woman and facilitate rapid self-healing by brushing away congestion in her energy system and relieving trauma immediately after her accident. If this swift healing is possible in one human being, it is possible in others. We need to do Healing Touch and let the results stand for themselves. It would be a disregard for human life not to do it.

BETTE: Do medical doctors request that you treat their patients?

JANET: Most of the time the invitation comes from the client and is offered with the approval of the doctor or hospital staff. In some situations we do in-hospital work with patients pre-operatively and post-operatively, and frequently in neonatal intensive care for preemies. Some hospitals in the United States and Canada have adopted Healing Touch as part of nursing practice. A common trend these days is that many hospitals want everyone on their staff to be able to do the Healing Touch. The US Navy has also been working with us because Healing Touch, along with first aid, has proven to be so beneficial in times of emergency. They arc pleased with the calming effect of the Healing Touch, and how it helps control bleeding. I personally would never have any procedure done without receiving Healing Touch.

BETTE: How long does it take to learn Healing Touch?

JANET: It takes a student about 2 years to complete the 120 classroom hours plus homework that are covered in 5 courses. We have over 600 certified Healing Touch practitioners. Healing Touch classes are offered here in Denver at our main office. Twelve tables fit comfortably in the classroom and 35 students can be seated. There are 2 treatment rooms for individual work on clients. People from all over the world come to Denver to learn Healing Touch.

BETTE: Do you teach Healing Touch in other cities besides Lakewood, Colorado?

JANET: Yes, I do, along with over 100 other certified instructors. Most of the time we are out teaching in communities. We run about 30 workshops a weekend, domestically and overseas. My primary focus is on training people to become instructors or practitioners who will take the program out into the world. Our international program is growing rapidly. Healing Touch is in Australia, the Netherlands, every province in Canada, South Africa and in Great Britain. Recently, Healing Touch was presented at the International Congress of Nursing, held in Vancouver, BC, Canada. Many foreign delegates asked us to discuss teaching Healing Touch in their countries. We expect that it won't be long before Healing Touch will be taught all over the world.

BETTE: Does Healing Touch work on animals?

JANET: It does. We have a whole department that teaches students how to work on horses, dogs and cats.

BETTE: Have you worked in any other profession besides nursing?

JANET: No. I went to nursing school at the University of Colorado after I graduated from high school. I always knew that I wanted to be a nurse. I am a healer, drawn to wellness.

BETTE: How did you start the Healing Touch program?

JANET: Years ago I took a Therapeutic Touch workshop taught by a former student of Dr. Krieger's. It was one of those momentous events for me. When I felt the energy field, I recognized that I had felt it before. And I knew that this was the kind of healing that I wanted to do for the rest of my life. I began studying with Dr. Krieger, Rev. Noel, and other distinguished healers. I went to the Edgar Cayce A.R.E. Center in Virginia Beach and took healing courses with Dora Kunz and Ethel Lombardi, both considered masters in their field. I studied the Edgar Cayce introductory course. And I got really good exposure on the work of many major healers. Everything I learned about energetic healing I taught to my continuing education nursing students at Denver's Red Rocks Community College. I have been an instructor there for over 20 years. In 1985 I opened a small office in Denver where I treated clients with a combination of therapeutic energy techniques not then named as Healing Touch. In 1990 the American Holistic Nurses Association approved the development of an energy-based program into a multilevel educational course for nurses and health care professionals.

BETTE: To how many nurses have you taught Healing Touch?

JANET: Since the beginning when the Healing Touch core faculty of nurses developed the program, our instructors have taught over 50,000 students. Last year, I was invited back to the A.R.E. to teach Healing Touch. I chuckled to myself because I had gone full circle. I was giving back all that I had learned years ago at the A.R.E., from many other healers, along with energy healing techniques I had developed myself.

....

For Further Information About Healing Touch Contact:

Colorado Center For Healing Touch
198 Union Boulevard
Suite 204
Lakewood, Colorado 80228
303-989-0581

....

RECOMMENDED READING

LIGHT EMERGING
Barbara Brennan
Bantam Books, 1993

WHEELS OF LIGHT:
Chakras, Auras, and the
Healing Energy of the Body
Roselyn Bruyere
Simon & Schuster, 1994

MINDING THE BODY,
MENDING THE MIND
Joan Borysenko,
Addison-Wesley
Publishing Co., Inc., 1987

....

I see myself as a healer of healers and a teacher of teachers.
My purpose in life, as I have come to understand it, is to
provide educational opportunities for people to learn
the work that I do and the work of other healers,
by teaching teachers who teach others.

Janet Mentgen, RN, BSN, CHTP, CHTI,
Developer of Healing Touch

2

SPIRITUALITY, RELIGION, PRAYER AND MEDICINE
The Doctor - Patient Connection

....

...prayer is the making of one's conscious self more in attune with the spiritual forces that may manifest in a material world... Prayer is the concerted effort of the physical consciousness to become attuned to the consciousness of the Creator, either collectively or individually.

EDGAR CAYCE
Reading 281-13

Our genetic blueprint has made believing in an Infinite Absolute part of our nature...To counter (our) fundamental angst humans are ...wired for God.

Herbert Benson, MD
Associate Professor of Medicine,
Harvard Medical School

...controlled studies show that prayer has positive effects even when tested under stringent conditions in double-blind studies in hospitals and laboratories. These studies involved not only humans but non--humans as well...One hundred-thirty-one studies later, I concluded this is one of the best kept secrets in modern medicine.

Larry Dossey, MD
From: *HEALING WORDS*

....

SPIRITUALITY, RELIGION, PRAYER AND MEDICINE
The Doctor - Patient Connection

Medical schools and residency training programs are teaching courses that pay deference to the link between spirituality, and/or religious faith, and prayer and the healing of body, mind, emotions, and spirit. Suspicion and rancor has traditionally existed for over 200 years between science schooled doctors and religion. But a shift in consciousness has taken place, largely rooted in approximately 800 of the 1200 scientific studies published in respected peer-reviewed journals, indicating that spirituality, faith, religious beliefs and prayer work like medication for the body, mind, emotions and spirit. "These factors seem to account for faster healing after accidents or injuries, a feeling of general well-being and longer lives," says Dr. Harold G. Koenig, founder of the Center for the Study of Religion/Spirituality and Health at Duke University Medical Center, Durham, NC.

Spirituality is defined as a pathway to finding meaningful purpose in life through higher consciousness, mercy, love, faith, insight, empathy and divination. Religion, on the other hand, is a set of doctrines and cultural practices edifying one's spirituality. Religion, Spirituality and Medicine courses are teaching compassionate and efficacious approaches for confronting a patient's chronic ill health and stressful circumstances fraught with hopelessness. Instructors enlighten medical students and residents on the art of beneficent listening to a patient's apprehensions, hopes, values, ideals, life purpose and other spiritual philosophies expressed in religious and/or spiritual convictions, prayer, conceptions of God or a Higher Power, and other sacred principles held close to the patient's and doctor's heart.

"Prayer (done at a distance, or near the person being prayed for, by another person, for someone they know or do not know) even works for agnostics," says Herbert Benson, MD, Associate Professor of Medicine, Harvard Medical School. Evidence also exists about the positive effects of meditation on people suffering from many conditions including hypertension, grief, worry and infertility.

Dr. Benson maintains that 60% of doctors visits are for stress-related ailments that could be alleviated with meditation and prayer. These factors are responsible for activating the "Relaxation Response" which lowers heart rate, respiration and blood pressure. Benson's best-selling 1975 book *The Relaxation Response* covers the subject in depth. But cynics cite the cause of physiological corrections as the "placebo effect", the ability to self-heal through strong belief, even if the medicinal remedy is only a "sugar pill". However, Benson believes, "Most of the history of medicine is the history of the placebo effect, which is remembered wellness." He asserts that faith in the healing power of a medical therapy is instrumental in successfully treating 60% - 90% of the most common medical problems.

At Harvard Medical School's Mind/Body Medical Institute, a Spirituality and Healing Conference held in Denver, Colorado, March, 2000, Dr. Benson said: "It is likely that our patients believe in religious or secular spirituality. Belief needs to be combined with medicine and surgery for healing." Nevertheless, the June, 22, 2000 issue of *New England Journal of Medicine* reported a backlash to this trend by nine researchers and chaplains at Columbia University College of Physicians and Surgeons, New York City. Their studies concluded that no substantial validation correlates religion with health, and the studies that do, were based on "...limited, narrowly focused and methodologically flawed research..." which did not make a distinction between Quaker meetings and Roman Catholic masses. It also did not account for tension and disturbance experienced when people convert to other religions over family disapproval. Cautioning against doctors prescribing religion, they stated: "Religion does not need science to justify its existence or appeal."

The John Templeton Foundation is a nonprofit organization founded in 1987 by financier Sir John Templeton. The mission of the Foundation is to pursue new insights at the boundary between theology and science. This is to be accomplished through a rigorous, open minded and empirically focused methodology, drawing together talented representatives from a wide spectrum of fields of expertise. Using the "humble approach", the Foundation typically seeks to focus the methods and resources of scientific inquiry on topical areas which have spiritual and theological significance. This ranges across the disciplines from cosmology to health care. The Foundation also recognizes the importance of character in a free society and supports a broad spectrum of programs, publications and studies that promote character education from childhood through young adulthood. The goal is to encourage schools and colleges to reinforce such positive values as honesty, compassion, self-discipline, and respect, and to foster widespread conversations about character development and values. The "Templeton Prize for Progress in Religion" is given each year for extraordinary originality in advancing the world's understanding of God or spirituality. First awarded in 1973, past recipients include Mother Teresa of Calcutta, Lord Jakobovits, Chief Rabbi of Great Britain, Rev. Billy Graham, Aleksandr Solzhenitsyn and Pandurang Shastri Athavale. Currently worth over one-million dollars, the Templeton Prize is purposefully larger than the Nobel Prize in order to suggest that progress in religion is more important than any other area of human endeavor.

Templeton grant programs are extremely competitive. The competition bestows seven $100,000 grants for research and writing on the constructive engagement of science and religion. This prompted three-hundred-seventy-seven letters-of-inquiry and resumes to be submitted in January, 1999. Administered by Dr. William Grassie and Dr. Christine Gibian from the Philadelphia Center for Religion and Science on behalf of the John Templeton Foundation, a screening committee of twelve experts read initial proposals and selected twenty-eight applicants to submit full-applications. After peer reviews by thirty scholars from a variety of academic disciplines and religious perspectives, the final decision was made by three widely respected judges: Dr. Philip Hefner, a professor at Chicago Lutheran Seminary and editor of *Zygon: A Journal of Religion and Science*; Rev. Dr. John Polkinghorne, past president and now Fellow of Queens College, Cambridge, England, and a Fellow of the Royal Society; and Dr. Lawrence Sullivan, Director of Harvard University's Center for the Study of World Religions. The following is a list is of the seven eminent scholars in religion and science who were each awarded grants of $100,000: (Institutional affiliations and proposed book titles are also noted.)

Philip Clayton, Ph.D., California State University, Sonoma, California, for:
The Emergence of Spirit: God Beyond Theism and Psychicalism;

William Dembski, Ph.D., the Discovery Institute's Center for the Renewal of Science and Culture, Irving, Texas, for:
Being as Communion: The Science and Metaphysics of Information;

Noah J. Efron, Ph.D., Bar Illan University, Israel, for:
Golem, God and Man:
Divine and Human in an Age of Biotechnology;

Niels Henrick Gregersen, University of Aarhus, Denmark, for:
Theology and the Sciences of Complexity;

David J. Krieger, Institute for Communication Research,
Meggen, Switzerland, for:
The Self-Organization of Meaning:
A New Paradigm for Science and Religion;

Michael Ruse, Ph.D., University of Guelph, Ontario, Canada, for:
Darwin and Design: Science, Philosophy and Religion;

Robert Joyn Russell, Ph.D., Center for Theology and
the Natural Sciences, Berkeley, California, for:
Time in Eternity:
Theology and Science in Mutual Interaction

The Templeton Foundation subsidized polls of doctors and health insurance administrators on the role of spirituality in healing. They also are a sponsor of the Harvard Medical School Mind/Body Medical Institute, which presents a seminar on spirituality and healing in medicine. In 1998, the Foundation backed investigative research on 1007 people to determine what Americans think about prayer and its effect on medical treatment. The outcome prompted Dr. Templeton to say: "The positive results from scientific analysis on the clinical benefits of prayer and belief on health, combined with a patient's desire to acknowledge their spirituality, have lead more and more physicians and health care professionals to seek education in this area, which, until recently, has been unavailable."

Since 1995, the John Templeton Foundation has funded medical schools for spirituality and medicine curricula. The program, directed by Dr. Christina Puchalski at the George Washington Institute for Spirituality and Health (www.gwish.org), recognizes model curricula in spirituality and health for undergraduate and residency programs in US medical schools. These awards are largely responsible for enabling medical schools to offer courses which emphasize compassionate care and respect for patient's spiritual and religious beliefs.

Christina M. Puchalski, MD has pioneered the development of numerous medical school educational spirituality/medicine curriculum for undergraduate, graduate and post-graduate residency programs, as well as classes for practicing doctors. Before going to medical school, she was a research scientist at the National Institutes for Health (NIH). Always interested in medicine and clinical care, she often went to patient case presentations at the clinical center of NIH. She also did volunteer work at the Maryland State Mental Institution, Maryland State Mental Hospital. "I saw that illness causes people to question the very essence of who they are and provokes very deep spiritual searches," says Puchalski. "And I realized how much people need to be supported through this by their physicians."

When she went to medical school, Puchalski was amazed to discover that they didn't have classes on grief, end of life care, or spirituality. In 1992, when she was a second year medical student at George Washington University, she developed a course on these subjects with the sanction of the school faculty. A few years later George Washington School of Medicine, and other medical schools in the country, changed their curriculum to include more emphasis on whole patient care rather than the disease centered approach. "Our courses naturally fit into the whole patient care model," says Puchalski. "Patient's are not just their illnesses, they are cultural, spiritual, emotional, mental and physical components of their whole being."

Shortly after graduating from medical school, Puchalski became the director of the John Templeton Awards Programs for Curricular Development in Spirituality and Health. The courses that she has created emphasize communication skills between physician and patient concerning a patient's issues about their health and death and dying. Puchalski has developed a tool called "FICA: A Spiritual History". As part of the routine patient history, "...we teach students how to obtain a cultural history to see how religious, spiritual and cultural beliefs might impact health care decision making." Students are taught how to engage with patients on the spiritual level. This is a way for compassionate presence to occur, with the physicians full support, in loving service, of another human being.

Puchalski views spirituality as a person's search for ultimate meaning in their life. Scientific data suggests that the role of spirituality in serious illness and end of life care is vital in how a person challenges, understands and finds deep significance in their suffering. "One of my cancer patients told me that her bout with terminal illness helped her live in the moment, and see life in a richer, fuller way."

For clinical purposes it is important to define spirituality broadly because how people find meaning in life varies. According to Puchalski, spirituality can be found in religion, or a relationship with a god or a higher power apart from religion. It can also be attained through kinship with others, or encountered in rationalism, humanism, music, art and other creative pursuits.

"Spiritual values are at the very root of a service profession, like being a physician," she says. The courses she developed encompass looking at the ethical aspects and boundaries of addressing spirituality as physicians in terms of what they can and cannot do. Understanding how and when to collaborate with chaplains, clergy and other spiritual leaders "...who are trained far more than we are in delivering spiritual care..." is a major part of the studies. Students learn that discussing spiritual issues with a patient, is patient centered and respectful, not an opportunity to proselytize or ridicule beliefs.

The course of study also examines the student's spirituality and how it can be nurtured to promote their well-being and possibly act as the foundation of their professional calling as a physician. "When students come to medical school they are often very idealistic and in touch with being of humane service to others," says Puchalski. But it becomes difficult to retain feelings of compassion with the rigors of medical school training "...long hours, time constraints and the technical training necessary to become a competent doctor." Classes encourage students to continue to be compassionate and of service to patients even in the midst of external pressures.

Currently, Puchalski's courses have a long term ongoing evaluation to study the effects of spirituality/medicine programs funded through the John Templeton Foundation. (For more information on these courses visit the George Washington Institute for Spirituality and Health website: www.gwish.org). Out of the 125 medical schools in the world, 75 of them are now teaching these courses. "Spirituality has always been looked upon as part of the healing process," says Puchalski. As technology advanced between the late 1800s and early 1900s there was a split between science and religion, with science considered the more rational discipline, because religion could not be proven through scientific method. "However, there is a recognition that when it comes to human suffering and how people cope with illness, death and dying, science does not have all the answers," points out Puchalski. "There is no amount of science or technology that can give us an absolute explanation as to why there is suffering and death."

In today's health care system, "...demands are made on doctors to see more patients in a briefer amount of time," she says. "But people don't want to be treated like a protocol or a disease entity. They want to be listened to, respected for their spiritual, religious, and cultural beliefs and treated like human beings by their physicians." Puchalski's spirituality and medicine classes give emphasis to these values as good patient care. There is increasing recognition, of the merits of this course of study, by the medical profession.

There are also medical schools that offer spirituality/medicine courses of study without a bequest from the Templeton Foundation. For example, at

Northeastern Ohio Universities College of Medicine (NEOUCOM), Lura Pethtel, M.Ed. in Higher Education and Counseling, and John D. Engel, Ph.D., Professor of Behavioral Sciences, teach: *Spirituality: The Doctor-Patient Connection*. The course is an elective through the Human Values in Medicine Program, Behavioral Sciences Department. The medical students, a culturally diverse group, work on distinguishing the breadth of spirituality from religion by discussing their own spirituality in class. "They learn how to 'hear' and honor the spirituality of others without the fear of getting mired in religious debate," Pethtel says.

During the first and second years, students become skilled in incorporating spiritual elements into patient encounters, when appropriate. Each student interviews at least three patients to obtain their spiritual history and spiritual issues. "During these interviews, students always comment that they felt a closer connection and an ease with the patient that wasn't there before," says Pethtel. "And patient's report feeling a mental and emotional boost. They are impressed with the doctor-patient experience." The course also includes a focus on the connection of religious beliefs to health care, coordinated and taught with chaplains from the NEOUCOM consortium hospitals.

The College President and Dean, Dr. Robert Blacklow, and Executive Associate Dean, John D. Engel, Ph.D., fostered the development of the course. They encouraged Pethtel, who had great interest in spirituality, and retired physician Peter O. Ways, MD to develop the course content. It is offered as a four year medical school elective, with first and second year students attending 5 sessions per year. The program is extended during the third and fourth years through a series of evening sessions covering a wide range of special topics such as: Spirituality of Children, Spiritual Issues in Caring for the Addicted Individual, and Spiritual Issues in Dying. Recently, taking a patient's spiritual history has become part of medical interviewing training required of all students in the first year of their education.

Opinions about Pethtel's and Engel's classes in Spirituality vary among clinical faculty. It ranges from faculty participation in the course, or expressed interest to do so, to refusal to be involved because of the belief that the course focuses on religious issues. "Among physicians, faculty and other caregivers there is little consensus as to the meaning of spirituality, with a prevailing reluctance not to be caught up in religious debate or proselytizing," says Pethtel.

"Many do not realize that when they ask how the patient's family is handling his/her illness, or how the illness has affected the patient's work and the rest of his/her life, they are asking spiritual questions."

The AnMed Family Practice Residency Program, Anderson, SC, is not subsidized by a Templeton grant. Nonetheless, they offer 3 to 4 medical students or residents a year the opportunity to elect to think and grow regarding faith issues with patients. Students are given tools to assess and respectfully work with their patient's spirituality by presenting key spirituality concepts including: healing and wholeness, mindfulness, faith, forgiveness, guilt and shame, prayer, tragedy and the power and limitations of the healer. They focus on clinical integration of these subjects with regard to pregnancy and childbirth, chronic pain, psychiatric illness, addiction and dependency disorders, disability and care of the dying. "Our intention is to equip physicians to be more sensitive to the religious and spiritual life of their patients. We believe in its salutary effects on a patient's well-being, physically, mentally, emotionally and spiritually," says Stuart Sprague, Ph.D., one of the course directors of the "Religion and Medicine" elective at the residency program. The residency maintains that physicians who use spiritual insights to fully understand their patients can more effectively diagnose their illness and prescribe appropriate treatment. Dr. Sprague was trained in graduate school, at the Southern Baptist Theological Seminary, in philosophy of religion. He taught the subject for 20 years, at Anderson College, Anderson, SC. He has been a faculty member in Family Medicine for the past 5 years, serving at the Anderson Family Practice Residency Program, Anderson, SC.

According to Sprague, the program is not a class, but rather a one month experience. It is unanimously supported by the residency program and can be a third or fourth year clerkship or elective rotation for residents in training who take spirituality very seriously. Many scientifically oriented members of the medical establishment are skeptical of non-empirical realities. They see abstract or spiritual endeavors as irrelevant to the scientific practice of medicine. Participating medical students and residents, however, report that clinical interaction between attending physicians and patients, journal writing, and reading and discussions with faculty about spirituality and religion, have a positive outcome on their formation as doctors. They become more aware of the impact of their spiritual values upon their clinical practice, and more sensitive to the need for inquiry and consideration about their patient's spiritual values. Although the program has not yet measured the patient's reaction to this experience, anecdotal reports indicate a decidedly affirmative evaluation from them.

H.E. Woodall, MD is a full-time Associate Professor teaching family medicine at the AnMed Family Practice Residency Program, Anderson, SC. He is also a course director of "Religion and Medicine", a residency elective. Dr. Woodall says that prayer, religion and spirituality do not easily lend themselves to dependable, and repeatable measurement, which is the cornerstone of scientific inquiry. "To acknowledge that faith matters and is active in healing, is to entertain that scientific inquiry is limited in revealing truths, and that our tools of measurement are incomplete. It takes a truly confident, honest scientist to admit awe and wonder in the connections between healing, prayer, religion and spirituality."

...above all, pray! Those who are about the body, use, rely upon the spiritual forces...Know that all strength, all healing of every nature is the changing of the vibrations from within - the attuning of the divine within the living tissue of a body to Creative Energies. This alone is healing. Whether it is accomplished by the use of drugs, the knife or whatnot, it is the attuning of the atomic structures of the living cellular force to its spiritual heritage...

EDGAR CAYCE
Reading 1967-1

Science is showing us how mind and body,
body and mind are inseparable.

Herbert Benson, MD
Behavioral Medicine Specialist,
Harvard University

....

RECOMMENDED READING

HEALING WORDS: THE POWER OF PRAYER
AND THE PRACTICE OF MEDICINE
Larry Dossey, MD
Harper Collins, 1993

HANDBOOK ON RELIGION AND HEALTH
Harold G. Koenig, MD and colleagues
Oxford University Press, 2000

FAITH, SPIRITUALITY
AND MEDICINE:
Toward The Making Of The Healing Practitioner
EE.King
Haworth Press, 2000

GIFTS OF HEALING
Hugh Lynn Cayce
A.R.E. Press, 1976

....

More things are wrought by prayer than this world dreams of.
Wherefore, let thy voice rise like a fountain for me night and day.

Alfred Lord Tennyson
From his poem: *Morte d'Arthur*

3

AROMATHERAPY
The Institute of Integrative Aromatherapy
Conversations With Laraine Kyle, MS, RN, CS, CMT

....

Odors - have the Life Everlasting about thee often, and ye will find whether as a sachet or as a liquid it will bring strengthening vibrations to the body.

EDGAR CAYCE
Reading T3416-001 F

....

Integrative Aromatherapy embraces the art, science and bio-energetics of the skilled use of essential oils for their positive effects in all aspects of life.

Laraine Kyle and Valerie Cooksley
IIA (Institute of Integrative Aromatherapy)
Co-Founders and Faculty

Laraine Kyle, MS, RN, CS, CMT, is a psychiatric clinical nurse specialist, certified massage therapist, licensed esthetician, teacher and co-founder of the National Association for Holistic Aromatherapy, Boulder, Colorado, a nationally accredited diploma program. She holds an international certification in Aromatherapy and has studied with many respected educators of Aromatherapy throughout the world. For more than 25 years, Kyle has continued her education in many body/mind/spirit systems of care including meditation, yoga, guided imagery, applied kinesiology and skin care. She supports the integration of

Aromatherapy in health care by providing quality products, education and consultation to health care professionals and laymen. Her training and consultation has empowered others to render loving care to "touch hungry" chronically ill patients in long-term health care settings with Aromatherapy and touch therapy techniques.

....

Also the odors which would make for the raising of the vibrations would be lavender and orris root...

EDGAR CAYCE
Reading T0379-003 F

....

Valerie Cooksley, RN was one of the first nurses in the United States to become certified in Oncology through the Oncology Nurses Society. Cooksley has worked at the high-end of cancer treatment, infectious diseases and out-patient care. Convinced that it is wisest to work with natural forces, Cooksley pursued studies in holistic health, Aromatherapy, botany, Ayurveda, homeopathy, bio-energetics, mind/body medicine and nutrition. She graduated from the Pacific and Atlantic Institutes of Aromatherapy and the International Training Program in Essential Oils/Advanced Studies, Purdue University. Presently, she is studying with Dr. Bruce Berkowsky, NMD, MH, HMC, and Dr. Joseph S. Puleo, HMC. Cooksley lectures to the public and health care professionals on Aromatherapy, botanical medicine, natural health care and stress management.

Cooksley and Kyle founded the Institute of Integrative Aromatherapy, Boulder, Colorado, in 1997. The school provides a comprehensive and integrative approach to Aromatherapy and holistic health. Cooksley's best-selling book *Aromatherapy: A Lifetime Guide to Healing With Essential Oils* is the most comprehensive text on the subject on the market today. Her latest book *Comforting Scents - Your Personal Aromatherapy Journal* encourages self-discovery and reflection through journal writing, fragrant prose and delighting in the rich and varied botanical essences that surround us.

...certain or definite odors produce those conditions ...that allay or stimulate the activity of portions of the system...

EDGAR CAYCE
Reading T1551-001 F

Aromatherapy is the skilled use of essential oils to maintain wellness physically, mentally, emotionally and spiritually. It ranges from deep and penetrating therapeutic action to extreme subtlety of fragrances on the psyche. Essential oils are highly concentrated aromatic plant essences, often 75 times more potent than the fruit, flower, leaf, bark, root, wood, seed or resin of derivation. Steam distillation is the most common way to extract essential oils from an aromatic plant. As the steam is forced through a vat of plant material, the oil glands of the plant are ruptured, releasing the volatile oils. Later, the oils separate from the floral water which results from recondensation of the steam. Floral waters, also known as hydrosols, such as rose and lavender are used in Aromatherapy and were also recommended in readings by Edgar Cayce.

To effect wellness, and encourage various states of mind, Aromatherapy requires 100% pure unadulterated essential oils of therapeutic quality. Preferably, the oils should be harvested from naturally occurring fields of trees, grasses, herbs or roots, as opposed to synthetic fragranced oils or adulterated oils of compromised quality.

....

HISTORY OF AROMATHERAPY

Aromatic plants, essential oils, floral waters and other aromatic extracts have been used for centuries by every major culture. Anthropologists speculate that primitive perfumery began with the burning of gums and resins for smudging and incense with aromatic plant material. Egyptian records of antiquity tell us how resins, balms and fragrant oils were used by priests, who were also doctors for mystical embalming ceremonies and ritual offerings to their gods. Some of the plant materials Dioscorides wrote about in his *Materia Medica*, 100 AD, mention many of the herbs and essential oils we use today including cardamom, cinnamon, myrrh, basil, fennel, frankincense, juniper, pine, rose, rosemary and thyme. There were many scented ointments and oils recognized by Dioscorides for their ability to convey physical and psychological benefits. He spoke of: bay laurel oils used to produce a trance-like state, rose, myrtle and coriander, respected for their aphrodisiac properties, and myrrh and marjoram used as sedatives. History also records the use of aromatic oils in China and India during the same period that Egypt used essences. Ayurvedic medicine has always applied aromatic oils with massage using Jasmine as a general tonic for the body, rose oil as an antidepressant and liver strengthener, and chamomile for headaches, dizziness and colds.

Distillation of essential oils is credited to the Persians in the 10th century, although there is evidence of distillation long before that by other ancient cultures. By the 16th century printed books on Aromatherapy were readily available. *La Philosophie Occulte*, 1531, by H.C. Agrippa, said: "*Perfumes, sacrifice and unctions exist and spread their odors everywhere; they open the portals of the elements and the heavens whereby man can glimpse through them the secrets of the Creator.*" By 1597, a German physician, Hieronymus Braunschweig wrote several books on essential oil distillation which went through hundreds of editions in every European language. He referenced 25 essential oils including rosemary, lavender, clove, cinnamon, myrrh and nutmeg. The role of micro-organisms in disease was recognized in the 1880s. By 1887, French physicians first recorded laboratory tests on the anti-bacterial properties of essential oils. These early tests resulted from observing a low incidence of tuberculosis in the flower growing districts of southern France. In 1888 a paper was published showing that micro-organisms of glandular and yellow fever were easily killed by active properties of oregano, Chinese cinnamon, angelica and geranium.

By the 19th century the role of the medical doctor was well established. In spite of regular use of essential oils, the medical profession became firmly fixed on isolating the active principles of natural substances. Chemical drugs were produced based on the identified "active ingredient" of the natural substance. However, it should be noted that the French and German medical profession maintained a close connection with the healing properties of botanicals. They did not experience the schism with botanical medicine that the United States did over the last 200 years.

In 1910, Rene Gattefosse discovered the healing properties of lavender after severely burning his hands in a laboratory explosion. He later used the wound healing and antiseptic properties of essential oils in the care of soldiers in military hospitals during WWI. Gattefosse coined the term "Aromatherapy" with the 1937 publication of his book of the same name. And, Dr. Jean Valnet, a French army surgeon, used essential oils in the treatment of war wounds during the French Indochina War. He wrote the book *Practice of Aromatherapy* which was translated into English in 1964.

Aromatherapy is now part of a new paradigm for cost effective natural healing, and for good reasons. The pleasurable fragrant world of essential oils has many therapeutic benefits. It awakens the senses to prevent the spread of bacterial infection, effectively stimulates the immune system and improves many skin conditions. Most essential oils are naturally antiseptic and purify the air we breathe while relaxing the body and mind.

Cayce prescribed scent for a variety of ailments ranging from nervous afflictions and bronchial catarrh to tuberculosis. In reading T0461-001, Cayce explains to a man suffering from a number of maladies, about the persuasive influence of color and odor: ***"As to the organs themselves, as indicated from the activity of the sensory system, we find disorders to the eyes; at times the ears roar or buzz; the tendency for colds or congestion to affect the body easily, and the general activity as of a nervous strain in the sensory activity - as in taste, smell, hearing, seeing, feeling. The body responds to many colors....,(and to) the varied effects of odors upon the body, and more so would it be were there normalcy in the activity."***

Some hospitals, hospices and nursing homes are now introducing Aromatherapy through skin care products and air diffusion. There are numerous aromatherapeutic remedies for chronic conditions such as fibromyalgia, arthritis, pain syndromes, Alzheimer's, stress related disorders and care needs of the dying. The use of essential oils runs the gamut, from aiding minor ailments such as aching feet treated with a few drops of peppermint oil in a foot bath, to alleviating chronic pain with rosemary or lemongrass.

In the book *Healthy Pleasures* by Robert Ornstein, Ph.D. and David Sobel, MD, the effects of aromatic stimuli on stress and depression are addressed. The book cites clinical research showing that a whiff of spiced apple fragrance modified the stress response by lowering blood pressure, decreasing respiration and pulse and relaxing muscles. One company now offers strawberry scented surgical masks to help calm patients under anesthesia. However, spiced apple and strawberry aromas are derived synthetically and not considered true Aromatherapy by aromatherapists.

The body, mind and spirit are effected by Aromatherapy on many levels, as indicated by Cayce in reading T1402-001: ***"Hence again, to the entity in this***

experience in dealing in things that influence the lives of peoples - as odors, as cosmetics, as flowers, as those things that, as it were, arouse the depth of the thinking; or again it may be said, to make that union of expression of the mind; the mind of the body and the mind of the soul - that are one, yet may be so far apart, as may be illustrated in that variation the entity has experienced in individuals in a varying mood - as ye would term."

Essential Oils are also regularly used for creating an environment of spiritual attunement. This was recommended by Cayce in reading 1616-1 for a woman requesting the outlining of a method for meditation: ***"Odors, - the essence of the red clover should be that chosen. The odors of sandalwood or orris and violet are well for these, when the entity meditates, create an environment for the entity."*** Sandlewood has a cooling and calming effect on the nervous system and can be used for agitated emotional states and sleeplessness.

Today, many nursing homes working with Alzheimer's patients have found that diffusing essential oils or spritzing diluted essential oils in water creates a relaxing environment. In small group settings, Alzheimer's patients are guided in sampling a variety of scents, resulting in memory recall and a noticeable increase in communication between residents. Using scent for prompting memory association of past life abilities, for application in the present incarnation, was indicated by Cayce in reading T0379-003: ***"Also the odors which would make for the raising of the vibrations would be lavender and orris root. For these were those of thy choice in the Temple of Sacrifice. They were also thy choice when thou didst walk with those who carried the spices to the tomb."***

Kyle has experienced lavender to be a fragrance of choice by many hospice patients, even when more exotic aromas have been available. In reading 274-10, Edgar Cayce said that lavender is ***"...that which angels of light and mercy would bear the souls of men to a place of mercy and peace."*** Unless there is a respiratory sensitivity such as asthma, allergy or chronic congestive pulmonary disease, patients and their families are happy to have pleasant aromas brought into their environment. In hospice care, castor oil packs for constipation, mentioned many times in the Cayce readings, are used effectively in combination with sweet fennel, marjoram and black pepper essential oils.

USES OF ESSENTIAL OILS

Aromatherapy can be used as a topical application mixed with massage oils and lotions, inhaled via air dispersion, applied by compress or experienced through aromatic baths with the use of salts or other emulsifying agents. These applications of Aromatherapy can deeply penetrate, nourish, rejuvenate and soothe the skin. Through inhalation, aromatic molecules are absorbed via the nose and lungs, regulating, invigorating, refreshing, and relaxing physically and psycho-emotionally.

Our perception of smell is unique, with nerve receptors just beneath the brain, level with the bridge of the nose. When inhaled, aromatic molecules transport their vibrational message through the nasal passage. At this location they stimulate olfactory receptor sites, and trigger nerve messages to the limbic center brain which is believed to have evolved over 70-million years ago. The limbic system represents a complex area. It contains 34 structures and 53 pathways that stimulate physiological responses within the body via the nervous, endocrine or immune systems. It affects the sensations of pleasure, pain centers of the brain, emotions, memory, sleep, appetite and sex as illustrated in *Song of Solomon*, 4:13-16, the *Jerusalem Bible*:

How delicious is your love,
more delicious than wine!
How fragrant your perfumes,
more fragrant than all other spices!
The rarest essences are yours:
nard and saffron, calamus and cinnamon,
with all the incense-bearing trees;
myrrh and aloes, with the subtlest odors.
Fountain that makes the gardens fertile,
well of living water, streams
flowing down from Lebanon.
Awake, north wind,
come, wind of the south!
Breathe over my garden,
to spread its sweet smell around.

and from Exodus 30:34:

*Take unto thee sweet spices, stacte, and onlycha and gallbanuum;
these sweet spices with pure Frankicense: of each shall there be a weight:
And thou shalt make it a perfume, a confection after the art of the
apothecary, tempered together, pure and holy.*

Numerous ancient cultures used Aromatherapy and incense for religious contemplation and medicinal purposes. Many of these very old traditions are in use today, like the use of incense for ceremony in the Catholic church. Laraine Kyle, co-director of the Institute of Integrative Aromatherapy, once interviewed Yeshe Dondon, the personal physician to the Dalai Lama, regarding the Tibetan tradition for the use of incense. Dondon described smudging himself with incense at dawn, noon and dusk to dispel negative environmental influences and to magnetize positive energy. In the mid-1980s while on a Buddhist pilgrimage to Japan, Kyle was introduced to the traditional Japanese Koh-do ceremony (an incense game of remembering scents of fine aloe wood) while she was at the Shoyeido Incense Shop founded 280 years ago. When she returned to America she hosted the lineage heir of the Shino School of Incense and a group of Japanese Koh-do practitioners who performed the Koh-do ceremony in Boulder and Denver, Colorado.

Aromatherapists, from ancient times to the present understand and respect the statement made 2,500 years ago by Hippocrates, the "Father of Modern Medicine". He said: *"A key to good health rests upon taking a daily aromatic bath and scented massage."* Laraine Kyle and her partner Valerie Cooksley were mindful of these words when they launched their Aromatherapy school in Boulder, Colorado. The Institute of Integrative Aromatherapy offers a certificate program and correspondence courses which have been welcomed by holistic health care practitioners and laymen.

Look to the perfumes of flowers and of nature for peace of mind and joy of life.

WANG WEI, 8th Century, AD

CONVERSATION BETWEEN BETTE MARGOLIS AND LARAINE KYLE

I first became aware of the Institute of Integrative Aromatherapy, Boulder, Colorado, when I read about the school in Nexus Magazine, Boulder, Colorado's holistic journal. The Institute offers a certificate course and community workshops in the theory and clinical practice of Aromatherapy. I was curious and wanted to know more, so I contacted Laraine Kyle, co-founder of the Institute.

She told me that the Aromatherapy course is offered in a workshop format of five 2-day trainings, and by distance learning. Studies include the uses of 50 essential oils which can be integrated with other holistic healing methods such as massage, acupressure and imagery for a broad range of physical, psycho-emotional and spiritual conditions. The use of essential oils is considered for all stages of life, from birth to death, in relation to numerous psychological and physical conditions.

The course of study also includes the history of Aromatherapy, extraction methods, safety considerations, the science of Aromatherapy, examination of the botany of aromatic plants and the chemistry of essential oils. Also analyzed are: basic anatomy and physiology of the skin, olfaction, lymph systems, pain relief, skin care, infection, wound healing, women's care including pregnancy and childbirth, detoxification, first aid and home health, essential oils for specialty populations such as cancer, hospice, AIDS, and fibromyalgia patients, and the examination of a variety of carrier oils - oils and lotions that dilute the concentrated essential oils to a usable and safe concentration.

"Carriers" that Cayce suggested are: castor oil, witch hazel, olive oil, and lanolin. Kyle does not recommend the latter for skin care because it tends to clog skin pores, diminishing the breathability of the skin and its ability to excrete waste. However, lanolin is effective for skin care by protecting the skin from moisture and inclement weather.

SAFETY CONSIDERATIONS

Safety-in-use considerations are examined in the Institute of Integrative Aromatherapy course. Not all essential oils that are distilled are safe for personal or professional use. Those that are chemically toxic to the nervous system, kidneys and liver, such as pennyroyal, wormwood, wintergreen, sassafras and camphor, are not generally available to the public. Citrus essential oils, such as lemon, orange, bergamot and angelica root are phototoxic, causing an excessive reaction to sunlight that results in rapid tanning or burning of the skin. Some asthma sufferers can be triggered by Aromatherapy. But essential oils can be used on sinus reflex points on the feet and pads of the toes with minimal risk of inhalation. People who are allergic to perfumes should not assume they are also allergic to essential oils. Fragrance allergies often result from sensitivities to the alcohol base, chemical extenders and stabilizers that are found in perfumes and not from essential oils per se. It is important to know the Latin botanical names of essential oils as various plant species reflect varying chemical composition. Evidence of pregnancy, seizure disorder or high blood pressure are other considerations when selecting essential oils or deciding on the dilution of a blend.

A few essential oils recommended by Cayce have cautioned uses according to current Aromatherapy information. Sassafras and yellow camphor can be lethal if not used appropriately or ingested accidentally by children. Sassafras has traditionally been used for treating high blood pressure, rheumatism, gout, arthritis, kidney, and skin problems, and by the food flavorings industry in toothpaste, mouthwash and natural root beer. Edgar Cayce recommended sassafras for the care of fractures, sprains, backache and bruises. However, the chemical constituent safrole, present in sassafras at 85 - 90%, has been identified as carcinogenic in animal research. Large doses of sassafras oil can cause fatty changes in the liver and kidneys and through accumulation in the body may cause cancer of the liver, esophagus or kidneys. Safrole was banned as a food additive by the FDA in 1961, including its use in the production of natural root beer. The International Fragrance Research Association recommends that safrole containing essential oils not be used in fragrance, and that sassafras oil should not be made available to the public without clear warnings of its carcinogenic potential and need for extreme dilution.

Throughout the IIA course students receive over 200 pages of teaching materials. The requisite textbooks are: *Aromatherapy: A Lifetime Guide To Healing With Essential Oils*, by Cooksley, *Aromatherapy: The Complete Guide To Aromatherapy*, by Battaglia, *Natural Home Health Care Using Essential Oils*, by Penoel, and *The Gift of Touch*, by Rose. Blending supplies are provided for course blending practicums included in the training. A theme paper on specialty topics of interest is required, which gives the student an opportunity to research an aspect of Aromatherapy in depth. Kyle cited examples of theme papers including: *Skin Care for High Altitude Climate, Pregnancy and Childbirth, Chakra Uses* and the *Integration of Aromatherapy for Hospice and Neurotrauma Patients.* Students conduct 20 case assessments, formulate an Aromatherapy intervention, and recommend ways to evaluate the outcome, as well as research 2 essential oils in depth. The curriculum is approved for educational contact hours for nurses and massage therapists.

A SAMPLE AROMATHERAPY GUIDELINE

An Aromatherapy guideline begins by defining the problem to be considered, such as stress and anxiety. In a sample guideline it was reported that stress is a normal part of life and can be used positively to encourage peak performance, goal achievement and creativity. However, if one is under pressure for an extended time, the accumulative impact of stress can lead to frustration, irritability and stress related illnesses. Stress is recognized as one of the major conditions affecting health in modern society. Factors relating to stress can be mental, physical, environmental and chemical, such as junk food, drugs, and pollution. Sustained stress often results in a host of health concerns including fatigue, headaches, food cravings, depression, anxiety, irritability, indigestion, insomnia and irregular heartbeat. The goal for dealing with stress is: improved coping with stresses of every day life, restoring and sustaining positive emotions and encouraging a balanced body-mind relationship.

The International Fragrance and Flavor (IFF) organization has conducted studies in which they have found that orange blossom, orange and other citrus scents reduce stress and depression. Other supportive data includes 1973 research by Dr. Paolo Rovesti who used essential oils to treat depressed and anxious patients. He found fragrances considered "green" or "herbal", like lavender, marjoram, rose and cypress, useful in treating depressed and anxious patients. And in an issue of the *British Journal of Occupational Therapy*, 1992, they cited the use of Aromatherapy in promoting health and well-being through massage, inhalation, baths, compresses, creams and lotions. The article offered a list of potential effects including: decrease in stress, sedation, relief of depression, promoting alertness and facilitating interaction and communication.

Essential oils promoting relaxation are: Roman chamomile, sweet marjoram, geranium, lavender and neroli (orange blossom). Some essential oils, such as lavender and geranium, have adaptogenic or balancing properties. When used in moderation they can have either relaxant or stimulant effect, dependent on individual need. The recommended methods for application through room diffusion, compress and massage, using scented oils and lotions, bath and direct inhalation from an essential oil bottle or tissue with an essential oil applied, emphasize the importance of choosing therapeutic grade essential oils produced from a known botanical source rather than synthetic fragrances.

Essential oils may be blended in various combinations and added to a carrier base. For example, a massage blend is generally made with about 15 drops of an essential oil to one ounce of an unscented lotion or vegetable oil of choice such as grapeseed, apricot kernel or almond oil. A compress can be used with 4 or 5 drops of essential oil blended with a vegetable oil and castor oil. A bath preparation can be made with 6 drops of essential oils in 1/2-a-cup of Epsom salts.

An effective balancing daytime blend can be made with lavender, geranium and a hint of lemon. A relaxing bedtime bath blend can be produced with lavender, marjoram and ylang ylang. A soothing evening diffuser blend can be created with 2-parts of lavender to 1-part orange with a hint of chamomile. Other holistic interventions that counter stress include reevaluating one's workload, fresh air exercises, yoga, meditation, deep breathing, visualization, music, and a balanced diet excluding sugar, processed foods, and omitting stimulants such as caffeine and nicotine.

Oil of lavender, when made buy passing flowers through
a glass alembic [when distilled], surpasses all other perfumes.

Dioscorides

Lavendula: these flowers are the parts used;
they are good against all disorders
of the head and nerves.

From: *THE FAMILY HERBAL*
Sir John Hill, MD, 1912

LAVENDER SUMMARY

Kyle provided an example of a summary on the essential oil of lavender which is steam distilled from the flowering tops and some leaves. Its place of origin was the Mediterranean area and is now cultivated mainly in France, Spain, England, Bulgaria and Tasmania. There are many varieties of lavender, such as lavandin (Lavendula x intermedia), a hybrid plant developed by crossing true lavender with spike lavender. Lavender is described as an evergreen woody shrub up to one meter tall, with pale green linear leaves and violet-blue flowers. The entire plant is highly aromatic with a sweet floral scent and herbaceous, balsamic woody undertones. The color of lavender oil can be clear or have a yellowish green tint.

Since ancient times, lavender has been a popular fragrance, valued in antiquity by Egyptians and Turks for its clean fresh scent. An infusion of lavender flowers in hot water was one of the earliest methods of use, which was applied externally as an aromatic "wash" or taken orally for various ailments. Arab women also used lavender oil as a hair treatment.

The Romans used lavender to fragrance their bath water and it is believed that the name stems from the Latin *lavare* - to wash. Compresses were made from infusions for their reputed antispasmodic action on internal organs. An infused oil made by macerating the flowers in hot animal fats or vegetable oil has long been used for anti-inflammatory and healing properties, such as healing skin damaged by overexposure to sun and wind. Lavender is non-toxic and is particularly used in conditions where a strong emotional component such as anxiety or fear predominate. Very few people develop skin irritation when using Lavender. It has been tested with a 16% concentration on humans with normal skin without adverse reactions.

AROMATHERAPY EDUCATION AND SUGGESTED OILS

"Can anyone attend classes?" I asked. I learned that the curriculum was primarily developed for nurses, massage therapists, estheticians and other holistic health care practitioners. There is also an in-depth home study course of more than 50 essential oils and aromatic extracts, botanical and chemical data, and skilled application techniques for a wide variety of bio-psycho-social-spiritual conditions. Some students without a health care background have taken the course to make Aromatherapy products for friends and family, as a hobby or to help chronic medical conditions. "Laymen without a background in anatomy and physiology have to study a bit more independently between classes," Kyle told me. Many students bring various health related skills such as nutrition, kinesiology, reflexology and herbology which are used to complement uses of essential oils whenever possible. Kyle stated that students are encouraged to reason out the skillful incorporation of essential oil application in daily life, once the various properties and applications of the essential oils are learned.

I asked Kyle if there were any Aromatherapy recipes for family health that I could try at home. She told me that health supporting and self comforting rituals are easily created with aromatics. And she advised exploring my personal response to various essential oil aromas. For example, Aromatherapy is used in scented pillows, candles, diffusers, special bath rituals, body brushing and skin exfoliation with medium-ground cornmeal and sea salt.; these ingredients can stimulate circulation, assist lymphatic drainage and remove dead skin cells as well as stimulate the growth of new skin cells. I learned that combining the use of Aromatherapy with massage and imagery is very supportive in working with rapid change, losses, recovery from addiction and for supporting personal development. I have tried a number of the following formulas, adapted from recommendations by Valerie Cooksley, with excellent results:

Muscle Relief Massage Oil: lavender 6 drops; rosemary 3 drops, juniper 2 drops, peppermint 2 drops with 1/2 ounce vegetable oil or lotion.

Serenity Blend: lavender 6 drops, bergamot 2 drops, ylang ylang 2 drops. Use with bath salts or add to 1 ounce distilled water in a spray bottle.

Headache Blend: lavender 10 drops, peppermint 5 drops, with 1/2 ounce vegetable oil or lotion carrier, 1 - 2 drops on each temple or inhale aroma from hands after rubbing them together briskly.

Morning Bath Ritual: Make a 1/2 ounce blend for daily use with cajeput 10 ml, eucalyptus 3 ml, black spruce 1 ml. Place 5 drops in the palm of hand and apply to one's moist body after leaving shower or bath, to underarms for deodorant use, or spread on the ball of the foot to energize and support the immune system for the day. (1 ml = 20 drops)

Spiritual Renewal: Consider frankincense, myrrh, spikenard, cypress, rose, neroli, lavender, helichrysum, or angelica essential oil with a specific intention or affirmation. Use with unscented body lotion, in the bath, spritzer, or as a daily personal fragrance.

COMMENTARIES FROM LARAINE KYLE

I have come to appreciate the many gifts Aromatherapy applications can provide in one's daily life. Health care is being redefined as we move into the 21st century, with the public encouraged to take an increased responsibility for health care maintenance. Many individuals are actively seeking information and products that will promote health, decrease the normal effects of aging and support the immune system. As new information, techniques and methodologies that support healing and wellness emerge, professionals involved in the field are examining the benefits that the public will hopefully embrace. Edgar Cayce, through many of his readings, provided an early framework for the uses of aromatic oils in self care.

Aromatherapy is currently used as a complementary health care modality in many countries including: the United States, England, Australia, Germany, France, New Zealand, South Africa and South America. Research in Aromatherapy is being conducted in clinical settings for the care of pain, anxiety, insomnia and other specific chronic conditions, and there is continuing need for such applied analysis. There are many quality Aromatherapy books available that guide readers in safe and skilled use of essential oils to support wellness and assist with alleviating minor ailments. However, to use Aromatherapy professionally, such as in nursing or a massage practice, a formal, recognized training in Aromatherapy is recommended. This will prepare the graduate for an optional US certification exam, sponsored by the Aromatherapy Registration Council and conducted by the National Testing Association. Successfully passing the exam allows the graduate to be included in a national registry of qualified aromatherapists.

....

Laraine Kyle can be contacted at:

The Institute of Integrative Aromatherapy
PO Box 19241
Boulder, Colorado 80308
Phone: 303-545-2002
or 888-282-2002

Valerie Cooksley can be reached at:

Phone: 425 - 557-0805
or 877-363-3422
Website: www.Aroma-RN.com

Food nourishes the body,
but flowers heal the soul.

OLD PROVERB

It will be found that the odors of henna,
with tolu and myrrh, create an influence of ease...

EDGAR CAYCE
Reading 1580-1 (25)

RECOMMENDED READING

AROMATHERAPY:
A Lifetime Guide To Healing With Essential Oils
Valerie Cooksley
Prentice Hall, 1996

THE ENCYCLOPEDIA OF ESSENTIAL OILS
Julia Lawless
Thorsons, Element, 1992

AROMATHERAPY FOR HEALING THE SPIRIT
Gabriel Mojay
Gaia (UK), 1996

AROMATHERAPY FOR HEALTH PROFESSIONALS
Shirley Price
Churchill Livingstone, 1995

For all its ancient origins, Aromatherapy in its modern form is still in its infancy! May the infant grow and thrive, and take its place among other forms of holistic medicine.

Patricia Davis,
Director of the
London School of Aromatherpy

AROMATHERAPY ORGANIZATIONS AND PUBLICATIONS

Aromatherapy Registration Council
c/o Professional Testing Corporation
1350 Broadway, 17th Floor
New York, NY 10018
(212) 356-0660

National Association of Holistic Aromatherapy
Publishes a quarterly publication:
The Aromatherapy Journal
4509 Interlake Avenue N #233
Seattle, Washington 98103-6773
(206) 547-2164

The International Journal of Aromatherapy
Harcourt Publishers Ltd.
PO Box 156
Avenel, NJ 07001
1-877-839-7126

Aromatherapy Today
(Australian Journal)
c/o ATP Springfields
PO Box 4583
Shreveport, LA 71134
(318) 868-1194

[Flowers]...no matter whether they be in or out of season - are well to be oft about the body. The beauty, the aroma, the aliveness of same will make for vibrations that are most helpful, most beneficial.

EDGAR CAYCE
Reading T1877-001 F

4

ON DEATH AND DYING
Interview With Dr. Elisabeth Kubler-Ross, MD

....

...a death in the flesh is a birth into
the realm of another experience,
to those who have lived in such a manner
as not to be bound by earthly ties.

EDGAR CAYCE
Reading 2147-1

....

Death isn't even a word in many medical dictionaries.

Michael Rabow, Researcher

Elisabeth Kubler-Ross, MD is a prominent, highly regarded psychiatrist and author. She is respected by the medical community and people of all races, colors and creeds throughout the world as the foremost authority on the terminally ill, AIDS patients and loved ones who survive them. Born in Zurich, Switzerland, she graduated from the University of Zurich Medical School in 1957. Kubler-Ross became a famous psychiatrist despite the protests of her upper-middle class Swiss parents who expected her to follow the conventional standard of the day and settle down as a homemaker whose life revolved around the church. A year after completing medical school studies, she came to New York City where she was a Research Fellow at Manhattan State Hospital. She married Manny Ross, a medical doctor with whom she had two children, Kenneth and Barbara.

Her continued studies lead to a degree in Psychiatry and more than twenty-five honorary doctorates for her extraordinary accomplishments in her lifelong work with the dying. As a young practicing physician she was appalled by what she described as "...the standard cruel treatment of shunning dying patients and being dishonest with them...." Kubler-Ross made it a point, unlike her colleagues, to spend time in and outside the hospital, respectfully and empathetically listening to near-death patients pour their hearts out to her. They candidly shared their fears, angers, concerns and sorrows with her, and openly cried and grieved, all steps in reaching a peaceful acceptance of their impending transition. Kubler-Ross observed that by releasing despair, terminally ill patients healed themselves emotionally and spiritually. She began offering her acclaimed lectures to the medical community and public in which she presented dying patients who spoke about what they were going through. They also talked about things they might have done with their lives, and what they finally realized truly mattered to them. It was a lesson not only about dying but also about the importance of living out one's purpose.

Her first book, *On Death and Dying* (1969) made Kubler-Ross an internationally celebrated personality. "My goal was to break through the layer of professional denial that prohibited patients from airing their innermost concerns," she wrote. Twenty other books followed her first one. She transformed worldwide thinking about death and dying by defining the psychological processes of the five stages of death: "Denial and Isolation", "Anger", "Bargaining", "Depression" and "Acceptance". Bravely she opposed taboos about the dying and examined the effects of a loved one's death on family values and lifestyles. She offered sound and merciful methods for fearlessly accepting the end of life with dignity and tranquillity. Her compassionate guidance provided peace for families and friends coping with profound anguish over the dying. She clarified the serenity that awaits those who pass from life's earthly ties into the next state of being.

In the early 1970s she worked with a Reverend who was a hospital spiritual counselor. They interviewed over 20,000 people of different ages, cultures and religions who had gone through near-death experiences. They all described a painless, peaceful transition to a beautiful new world, and pleasurable encounters with the souls of loved ones who had passed on. One interview with a 12-year-old girl convinced Kubler-Ross that all she had heard about life after death was true. The child spoke of a remarkable meeting with her deceased brother, someone she did not even know existed because she had never been told that he died shortly before she was born. Kubler-Ross and the Reverend concluded that the near-death experiences of all the people they interviewed were so comparable that their anecdotes had to be authentic rather then hallucinations or just random events. Kubler-Ross' books have been translated into more than twenty-five languages and include: *To Live Until We Say Good-Bye, On Children and Death, AIDS the Ultimate Challenge, Wheel of Life,* an autobiography, which she says is her favorite of all her books, and her most recent book *Life Lessons*, a work she collaborated on with Dr. David Kessler, about the mysteries of life and living.

...[death] is only a transition - or [a passing] through God's other door...For, as we have given, that we see manifested in the material plane is but a shadow of that in the spiritual plane.

EDGAR CAYCE
Reading 5749-3

....

Should you shield the canyons from the windstorms,
you would never see the beauty of their carvings.

From: *ON DEATH AND DYING*
Elisabeth Kubler-Ross, MD

....

Interview With Elisabeth Kubler-Ross, MD

Dr. Elisabeth Kubler-Ross will not be coming back. She is convinced that after her transition through "God's other door", she will be dancing in heaven for eternity, cradled in the unconditional love of the Creator. This reward for an exceptional woman will be well-earned. Single-handedly, with relentless dedication, she has spent her life enlightening millions of people on the art of fearlessly embracing the final passage of life with serene dignity. People of all ages, cultures and creeds have unburdened their deep grief over the loss of loved ones through her sensitive guidance. Kubler-Ross' lifelong devotion to fighting for compassionate treatment of near-death and AIDS patients, never wavered in the face of many heroic uphill battles she has confronted. It is her enormous strength of character and courage of her convictions that has carried Kubler-Ross through discords concerning medical and theological controversy, and conflicts with individuals hostile to her humane and spiritual ideals. The 75-year-old psychiatrist, and twenty-time best-selling author of international renown, now faces one of her greatest physical, emotional, and spiritual challenges: full recovery from a series of many strokes, one of them major, which she suffered six years ago, causing her partial paralysis.

She was lying on a bed in her sitting room when I entered the door to her adobe home in Scottsdale, Arizona. I knocked loudly before entering as she had instructed me to do via the phone.

"Who's there?" she called out in her Swiss inflection.

"It's me, Bette Margolis, how are you today?" I answered.

"Hanging in there," she acknowledged.

Because her hands are somewhat gnarled, a side effect of multiple strokes, she greeted me with an extended finger saying "ET" as a symbol of the stretched out healing finger of Steven Spielberg's beloved Extraterrestrial. I touched her fingertip with mine and felt pangs of sorrow for her current state of health. To me, and to her many admirers throughout the world, this woman, small in stature, has always been bigger than life. But in that moment she appeared very vulnerable and I was taken aback. She is, after all, flesh and blood like the rest of us, subject to life's vicissitudes. Faithful to her characteristic feistiness, she refused my help and slowly made her way from her bed to a nearby armchair with the aid of her walker.

"Please get me some English Breakfast tea with a spoon full of sugar. And help yourself," she said.

"Do you have help?" I asked, placing the tea cups into the microwave.

"Two days a week; I don't need it anymore then that," her voice seemed stronger by many octaves. "And my son lives nearby."

"Were you treated at a hospital when you had your strokes?" I inquired as I stirred some sugar into the tea.

"I'm a doctor; I can take care of myself. And I had my spiritual healer, Joseph; he helped me," she explained. "What did I need a hospital for? To ring a bell for someone to bring me water? Hospitals don't make you well; healing comes from within."

"How long has it been since the strokes?"

"Six long tormenting years; I have been waiting for my death," she took a deep long breath. "Of course, death does not exist. It is only a transition from bondage of the physical body. Everything in life is temporary, but the soul and spirit live forever. I have no fear of death."

I brought her the tea. "Let's make a toast: "L'Chaim," I said. "That's Hebrew; it means "To life!" Kubler-Ross was married to a Jewish man, so I was certain she knew what L'Chaim meant. I placed the teacup on the table next to her armchair.

She smiled, " My children practice the Jewish faith."

I glanced around her sitting room. A photo of the smiling Dalai Lama sat at the center of a table at eye level from her armchair. Around it were other framed pictures of her children and grandchild, and one of her spiritual healer. Outside the window birds were busily eating from a feeder. "Would you like some lunch?" she asked. "Can you make a poached egg?"

"Only scrambled or sunny side up!" I informed her.

"Make mine scrambled, soft, very little butter, and two slices of toast," she directed. I was happy to do this for her - it appealed to the nurturer in me, and I instinctively wanted to mother her. The eggs turned out okay but the toast was a little too dark, although she did not complain.

After lunch, I quoted Edgar Cayce's wisdom as a prelude to the interview questions I had written on a piece of paper: ***"...make the world a better place because you have lived in it."*** 5392-1. "You have certainly done this with unique courage and style, Elisabeth," I said. "But you have experienced the dark night of your soul and have been very angry at God."

"Anger is good. Externalize the suffering. Yes, I have been very angry for many things that have happened. Arsonists burned my home on a 300 acre farm in rural Virginia. I created a healing center there. They burned my home down because of my plans to adopt black AIDS infected babies to care for at the healing center." She squeezed her nostrils closed with her fingertips to assert the stench of bigotry, ignorance and hatred.

"Were you able to salvage anything?" I quietly asked.

"Nothing. All of my personal belongings were turned to ashes. My heart, my soul, my life went up in flames. Everyone goes through hardships; it's supposed to make you stronger. I had to accept my losses - what else could I do? My life has never been easy. But how else would we know what peace is if we did not experience the opposite? If not for anger how would I know the ultimate goal of patience? "

"That's why you left Virginia?" I continued.

"My son kidnapped me," she said sounding exasperated. He brought me to Arizona where he lives.'

"An act of love, not malice," I reasoned. "He was, no doubt, fearful for you and only wanted to protect you."

She shook her head yes, but looked irritable. "It's hot here in the desert; I don't like it."

"What do you think love is, Elisabeth?"

"Being there and caring," she answered.

"You are angry about your health?" I asked.

"After traveling all over the world lecturing to at least 40,000 people about the transition between life and death, writing books about it to educate millions of people, and spending my life in service to patients to ease their suffering, I thought I would have been granted a kinder old age. Yes, I am very angry."

"How do you feel about assisted suicide in cases of terminal illness causing severe pain and suffering?"

"It is wrong. If it is carried out, the suicide victim will only come back to experience a much worse lot."

"Would you change the course of your life if you could?"

"No, not one thing. I accomplished what I came here to do. I knew my path before I entered this incarnation. I chose it and would travel the same road again if I had to. Even this dark night of my soul is part of my destiny."

"To what purpose?" I asked.

"For learning patience," she stated. "The more lessons we learn, good and bad, the more fully we live life."

"Would you marry the same man even though your marriage ended in divorce?"

"Yes, I would. But he adopted a completely different lifestyle in his old age. I could not go along with his new passion for collecting material possessions. Then he remarried someone almost the age of his own daughter. I feel as though God is laughing at me."

"Laugh back," I suggested. "Get well and have a great love affair." She chuckled heartily, patting her knees.

"Is there a particularly important life lesson you've learned?" I asked.

"I should have had more balance in my life. I did not play enough," she confessed. "I did not nurture my soul through self-love."

"What are your plans for having some fun in your life now and caring for your soul?"

"I'm leaving for Switzerland in July to visit my sisters; we're triplets you know. As a child it was a great struggle to find an identity of my own. My sisters and I were always treated as though we were one. But I found my identity as an adult. I'll be traveling to Switzerland with my children and granddaughter." Her facial expression became softer at the mention of her grandchild.

"How old is she?" I asked.

"Two. She's like me - feisty," she smiled.

"So, your granddaughter gives you joy! What else gives you peace?"

"Chocolate gives me peace," she quipped.

I took out a box of chocolate from my carryall. "I brought you some candy as a gift." She thanked me. "And I also brought you a copy of my children's book *A Heart Full of Love*." I gave her a brief synopsis of the book, "It's for children of divorce on the art of making peace with oneself and one's family and stepfamily."

"Have you read my children's book *Remember The Secret*?" she asked.

"I didn't know you wrote a children's book," I told her.

"It's a spiritual story meant to comfort children who are contending with the death of someone dear to them. Friendly angel guides - we all have them - help the children in the story understand that death is not a dreadful thing, and eventually they will be happily in heaven with the one they lost," she explained.

"I used to think of death as synonymous with the saddest of human experiences," I divulged. I told Kubler-Ross about the death of my infant sister who was born with her brain exposed due to a difficult instrument birth. She shook her head empathetically. When I told her that doctors kept the baby alive for several months to see how the human brain functioned, she said, "Awful!"

"I wish my parents had read your books to heal their misery instead of swallowing it," I said. "They suffered lifelong emotional scars because of the sadness they never released. Tell me, what could possibly have been the purpose of the baby's life and death?"

"The baby's soul did not need a lifetime for learning the wisdom that it came to acquire," she explained. "It learned what it came to attain, and could therefore return to God."

"You have worked with dying children of all ages. Are they better teachers about death than adults are?

"Yes, because they don't disguise their feelings like adults tend to do. All children intuitively know what the outcome of their illness will be. And they can tell you exactly what they need for making peace with themselves."

"Do you keep in touch with your patients?"

She motions to a stack of mail. "Certainly, but it's hard for me to answer the letters that I receive these days because the stroke has made it difficult to write."

"In *Death and Dying*, you wrote about a mystical experience you had with the soul and spirit of Mrs. Schwartz, one of your patients who had passed on.

Have you had other encounters like this?" I inquired.

"Hundreds," she answered matter-of-factly. "Anyone can if you are ready for it; if not, you will deny your mystical confrontations."

I read her some facts from the Journal of the American Medical Association. They recently reported that most doctors do not learn to treat the dying patient. The study, supported by the Robert Wood Johnson Foundation to educate MD's for better patient care at near-death, revealed that only 12 out of 50 medical textbooks contained helpful or any information at all about treating patients close to death; 29 texts had no information about care at the end of life; no mention of death was found in 71.8% of books on surgery; 70% of books on AIDS and infectious disease had nothing on death; and 61.9% of books on cancer had no information about death. Textbooks most likely to have information on the end of life were about family medicine, geriatrics, and psychiatry.

"It figures!" she commented.

"What else can be done to close the gap in humane and meaningful patient care at near-death and for the living who grieve for the dead?" I asked.

"The medical community has made some progress. In time they will learn."

"Are you continuing to work with patients despite your current state of health, Elisabeth?"

"Of course," she answered emphatically. "We are here to help heal one another, and to liberate our spirits and souls from the dark side of our natures which we all possess."

She lit up a cigarette and took a few puffs. "My doctors advised me to give up smoking and chocolate, too," she told me as she finished her cigarette. "But these are my small pleasures at this stage of my life."

Before I left, she asked me to move her walker, which was blocked by her bedside commode, to the front of her armchair. I honored her request. Slowly she made her way back to her bed and laid down. "ET," she whispered, and our fingertips touched, as I said goodbye.

....

Each entity enters materiality for a purpose.... What is the purpose of entering consciousness? That each phase of body, mind and soul may be to the glory of that Creative Force in which it moves and has its being.

EDGAR CAYCE
Reading 1947-3

....

RECOMMENDED READING

Books By Dr. Elisabeth Kubler-Ross:

LIFE LESSONS
Scribner, 2000

ON DEATH AND DYING
Simon & Schuster, 1969

DEATH:
The Final Stage of Growth
Simon & Schuster, 1997

THE WHEEL OF LIFE
A Memoir of Living and Dying
Simon & Schuster, 1987

LIVING WITH DEATH AND DYING
Simon & Schuster, 1997

TO LIVE UNTIL WE SAY GOODBYE
Simon & Schuster, 1997

ON CHILDREN AND DEATH
Simon & Schuster, 1997

QUESTIONS AND ANSWERS
ON DEATH AND DYING
Macmillan, 1974

AIDS:
The Ultimate Challenge
Simon & Schuster, 1997

ON LIFE AFTER DEATH
Celestial Arts Publishing Co., 1995

THE TUNNEL AND THE LIGHT
Essential Insights on Living and Dying
With a Letter to a Child With Cancer
Marlowe & Co., 1999

MORE RECOMMENDED READING

EDGAR CAYCE'S STORY OF THE SOUL
W.H. Church
A.R.E. Press, 1991

NO DEATH:
God's Other Door
Hugh Lynn Cayce and Edgar Cayce
A. R.E. Press, 1999

....

Contact Dr. Elisabeth Kubler-Ross at:

Phone: 480 - 488-8220
Website: www.elizabethkublerross.com

....

In that moment - as in birth, we have the beginning of an earthly sojourn, a little or long, as time may be - so the birth into the spiritual plane begins with the death in earth plane; merely the separation of the spiritual and soul forces from the earthly connections.

EDGAR CAYCE
Reading 900-19

....

5

COMMERCIAL BREAK:
The Complete Couch Potato's Guide to Fitness
Linda J. Buch and Seth Anne Snider-Copley

" A Book Review By Bette S. Margolis"

....

Regular exercise changes the body structurally and metabolically. The heart becomes stronger and pumps more blood with less effort, lung capacity increases, and muscles become more energy efficient. Exercise also helps us stay leaner, improves sleep patterns, alleviates constipation, retards bone mineral loss and greatly improves our outlook on life. With all the evidence, it is not difficult to concur with the readings: ***"Exercise is wonderful, and necessary - and little or few take as much as is needed, in a systematic manner."*** (283-1)

Eric Mein, MD
From: *KEYS TO HEALTH*

Linda J. Buch has a weekly fitness question/answer column in the Sunday Denver Post Lifestyles section. Buch is a personal fitness trainer for the past 15 years. She was a health and fitness consultant for the Rocky Mountain News, (Scripps-Howard) Denver, Colorado, and is the co-author of *COMMERCIAL BREAK: The Complete Couch Potato's Guide To Fitness* (Balance/Fitness Books, 1999).

Seth Anne Snider-Copley, co-author of *COMMERCIAL BREAK,* is a fitness trainer, exercise physiologist and registered kinesiotherapist. She deals with the body as it relates to movement, and integrates physical therapy with the central nervous system. With over 15 years of fitness and wellness experience in private and corporate sectors, Snider-Copley has worked with members of the US Alpine Special Teams, snowboarding team, Olympic Athletes and World Champions at Body Dynamics Health Studio and she is an aquatic exercise specialist for the Aquatic Exercise Association.

COMMERCIAL BREAK

Exercising the Easy Way
"A Book Review By Bette S. Margolis"

I am not and have never been a couch potato, but my good friend Annie is. She has pretty much given up on the idea of fitness because she says losing weight is a lost cause for her. Annie's angst about being overweight propelled her, like more than half of Americans, to head home from her high powered, high stress job, plop down on her soft couch, and tranquilize herself with a dinner of high calorie fast food and an evening of watching her favorite TV shows. Because I am her friend, I am concerned about her well-being, so I gave her a copy of wellness instructor's Linda Buch and Seth Anne Snider-Copley's book *COMMERCIAL BREAK: The Complete Couch Potatoes Guide to Fitness.* We found the book to be encouraging, easy, pleasant, often humorous, light reading, with charming illustrations and down to earth text, set in large type, that shared insights into the art of shedding pounds, without sweating, groaning, or collapsing in pain, to affect positive change for fitness. "And, our regimen for getting into shape never interferes with your favorite TV programs because we designed the exercises to be done during 3 minutes of TV commercial breaktime," say the authors.

The book is in agreement with Cayce's cautious approach to exercise: ***"To overexercise any portion (of the body) not in direct need of same, to the detriment of another, is to hinder rather than to assist...Use common sense. Use discretion."*** (283-1). *COMMERCIAL BREAK* also recommends consulting with a physician before initiating any new exercise program, even an easy one for couch potatoes.

"Now that's my kind of fitness program," Annie remarked, with peaked interest and high expectations. According to Buch and Snider-Copley, expectation is often a prediction of the future and contributes to making something happen. After consulting with her physician who heartily told her to "go for it", Annie followed through with *COMMERCIAL BREAK'S* "user-friendly" exercise and diet program. Results? Six months later, there's a whole new Annie, 35 lbs. lighter, and getting fitter every day, without interrupting even one of her favorite TV programs. And she's even graduated to taking outdoor walks and bike rides with no signs of TV withdrawal symptoms.

What impelled the authors of *COMMERCIAL BREAK* to write an effective program about fitness for couch potatoes? It was Surgeon General C. Everett

Koop's report on physical activity and health that was one of the catalysts for the authors. The report contained overwhelming statistics relating to obesity. It said that 500,000 Americans a year develop metabolic diseases related to poor diet, stress, inactivity and sedentary lifestyle. In fact, not exercising is equivalent to smoking a pack of cigarettes a day. Koop recommended significant dietary changes, and *"...accumulation of only 30 minutes or more of moderate intensity physical activity, over the course of most days of the week, to dramatically enhance wellness by bringing blood pressure down, reducing body fat and elevating energy and mood."*

Between work, kids, family schedules, meetings and personal obligations, Americans are working harder now than ever before," says Buch. "The most common excuse for choosing inactivity over improving physical fitness is: "I cannot squeeze one more thing into my busy schedule." Yet, Buch and Snider-Copley found that we normally relax by spending 4 hours a day watching TV. *COMMERCIAL BREAK*, guides readers in safe and progressive exercises, according to ability, from light to moderate intensity, during 10 - 12 minutes of total TV commercial break time. The authors determined that each break is approximately 2 minutes and 30 seconds long, with 6 to 8 product or service advertisements per break, and 10 - 12 minutes of commercial time during a half-hour sitcom. "We realized that a typical evening of TV viewing affords the average viewer 30 to 60 minutes of commercial break exercise time," says Buch and Snider-Copley.

Health professionals and physicians classify obesity as being over 30% of ideal body weight, a category that 55% of American adults and 50% of children fall into. Poor diet, stress and a sedentary lifestyle, are blamed as culprits. The author's prescription for combating sedentary lifestyle lies in a simple four-letter word: "MOVE!" They tell readers that with only moderate activity during 30 minutes of commercial TV breaks each day, 1000 calories per week, beyond normal expenditure can be burned, significantly improving overall health and relative fitness, and lowering the risk of sudden death.

COMMERCIAL BREAK clearly defines a comprehensive and prudent plan for couch potatoes to get into shape, incorporating five essential components: posture, balance, flexibility, strength and cardiovascular conditioning. "And you can even spread out the exercises, one for each part of the body, in 3 - 4 hours of TV viewing or over 7 days," the authors point out. You can watch the "Rosie O'Donnell Show" or "Oprah" during the day, exercise at commercial breaks, then pick up the kids, run errands, or attend meetings and finish exercising at night during commercial breaks of the "Evening News", "Seinfeld", "Home Improvement" or other favorite TV programs. "While it is important to exercise at your own pace, it is also essential for couch potatoes to try some of the recommended program daily," says Buch.

The book lists posture as the first component to an effective and prudent fitness program. Posture conveys confidence, vitality and structural integrity. Strong abdominal muscles and strong muscles in the upper, middle and lower back are essential for improving posture. "As a bonus, you will look slimmer and feel far more vital," the authors explain. Poor posture, on the other hand, can accentuate headaches, sciatica, shoulder tension, hip and knee pain and compression of the spine which squeezes internal organs, decreases lung capacity, constricts blood vessels and can be a cause of chronic neck and back pain.

Buch and Snider-Copley define good posture as: head erect and directly over shoulders, shoulders square but relaxed, mid-back straight, arms/hands fall naturally to side, abdomen does not protrude, hips level, slight curve in the lower back and knees relaxed with feet directly under the knees. During a TV commercial break, couch potatoes can correct posture in 3 simple steps:

1) Stand against a wall with arms hanging naturally at your sides, and head, heels, upper part of your butt and shoulders touching the wall; 2) lift arms away from your sides until they are spread straight out from your shoulders parallel to the floor; then, turn your arms so palms of hands are facing toward the ceiling; 3) return arms to sides while keeping palms faced away from you. Allow your hands to return to their natural position as you feel your shoulders pull back.

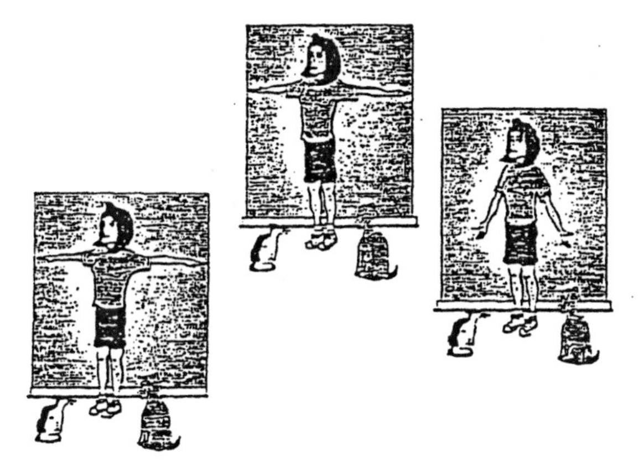

Yoga, Pilates, Swiss Ball, the Alexander Technique and the Feldenkrais Method are other alternative methods recommended by Buch and Snider-Copley for correcting poor posture and resultant chronic problems. Yoga, which is over 5000 years old, teaches breath, balance, flexibility and body alignment. Pilates uses spring-based equipment in all conceivable planes of motion. It involves precision, awareness, the use of breath to strengthen and lengthen muscles from the core to the extremities, and it opens up joints and releases tension. The Swiss

Ball (also known as the stability ball and the Fit Ball) promotes "active sitting" which stabilizes and strengthens the core muscles of the back and abdomen. The Alexander Technique teaches how to get rid of harmful tension in the body by reeducating the mind on movement, balance, support and coordination. The Feldenkrais Method educates the practitioner on awareness through movement for flexibility, coordination and relaxation. *(See End Of Chapter For Contact Information).*

"Posture and balance are interdependent because they rely on abdominal area and lower back muscles which are important for proper alignment and structural integrity," explain the authors. "As we age, balance often becomes impaired, resulting in injury." Buch and her co-author have devised simple exercises to quicken reaction time to the signal carried from brain to muscle. Balancing exercises in *COMMERCIAL BREAK* are divided into three levels. The first, the Beginner/Green Level, is for those who consider "cardiovascular exercise" a dash from the couch to the bathroom, and then to the refrigerator. The second, the Intermediate/Yellow Level, is utilized when the heart muscle is getting stronger. And the third, the Advanced/Blue Level, is for those who have graduated to performing exercise during every commercial break for two consecutive hours of TV programming.

Green Level balance exercise requires: standing next to a chair, without shoes, during the first commercial, lifting arms to sides, and with eyes closed, bringing arms together in front of you. If you can do the Green Level exercise without excessive wobbling or tipping, proceed to the next level. Yellow Level exercise, involves: standing on one foot, like a flamingo, next to a wall, stable chair or sofa, without shoes, and with closed eyes, keeping knees slightly bent. When you accomplish this exercise without excessive wobbling, tipping, or holding onto the wall, chair or sofa, it is time to go to the advanced Blue Level exercise. This requires a little walking space; with eyes closed and without shoes, take two steps forward, then two steps backwards.

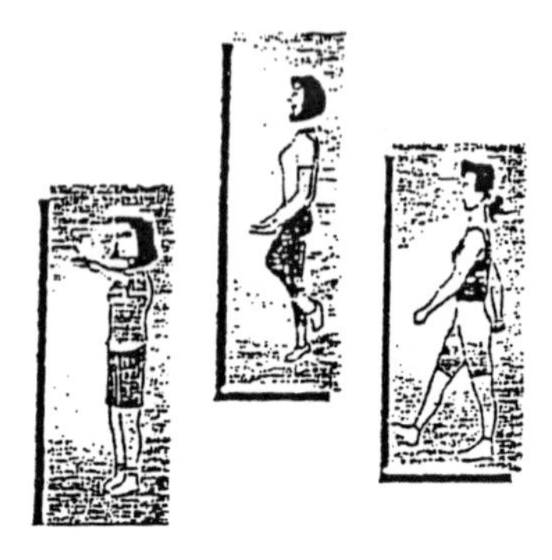

Buch and Snider-Copley suggest stretching daily, before and after exercise, to improve and uphold flexibility (the ability to move joints through their full range of motion) for resilient muscles and better muscle tone which is essential for fitness. Stretching keeps the joints lubricated when performing exercise and reduces the build-up of waste products such as lactic acid. Once bodily control has been mastered through various stretches, the body will be more responsive to

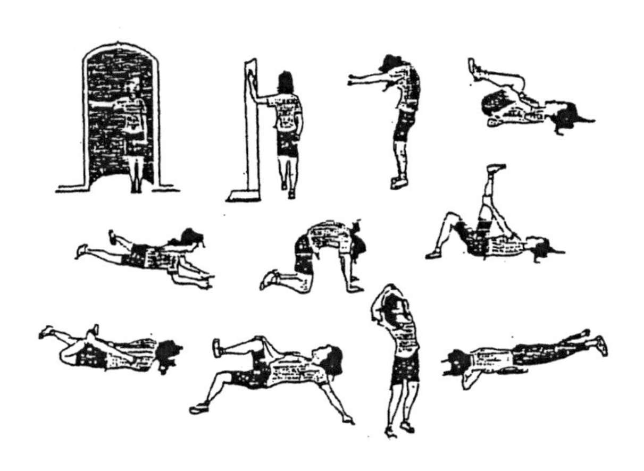

daily living activities. The authors explain that during sleep, the muscles and connective tissue shorten. After one wakes up the muscles with stretches, they return to their previous length. This assists with better muscle control and prepares the body for movements performed during the day that are more vigorous. Performing stretches before bedtime will relieve tight and fatigued muscles and encourage sound sleep.

COMMERCIAL BREAK includes drawings of couch potatoes exercising the right and wrong way to do stretches for the neck, chest, mid-back, back of shoulders, lower back, triceps (the back of arms), hips, butt, hamstrings (back of the leg between the butt and the knee), quadriceps (front of the leg between the hip and the knee) and abdominal muscles. Buch and Snider-Copley stress that stretching exercises should feel good. They are meant to be done twice, holding for 20 seconds or longer each time, which is about the length of many product TV commercials.

Muscle toning follows stretching. "Acquiring more muscle can mean the difference between aging gracefully or abruptly. After age 20, an inactive person loses about half-a-pound of muscle per year, " the authors explain. This is not the type of weight loss to celebrate because a pound of fat only burns 3 calories per pound per day, while a pound of muscle burns 50 calories per pound per day. This is why someone with more muscle mass has a higher metabolism and is able to keep fat off more easily than someone with high body fat. The more muscle you have, the more calories you require for the body's maintenance. Fueling the body properly to keep those hard-earned muscles happy and healthy is relatively simple. Foods that have a combination of carbohydrates and protein (essential amino acids) feed the muscles and help them perform physiologically at their peak. Another by-product of this is stronger bones which is particularly important for women. With age a woman's bone density often decreases, especially for inactive women.

"There is no such thing as "spot" reducing," state Buch and Snider-Copley. But their eight easy-to-follow strengthening exercises have been choreographed to progress smoothly from head-to-toe. Each exercise can be done during one commercial break, starting with the Green Level to increase muscle. All three levels, Green, Yellow and Blue, are designed for increasing muscle and improving muscle tone.

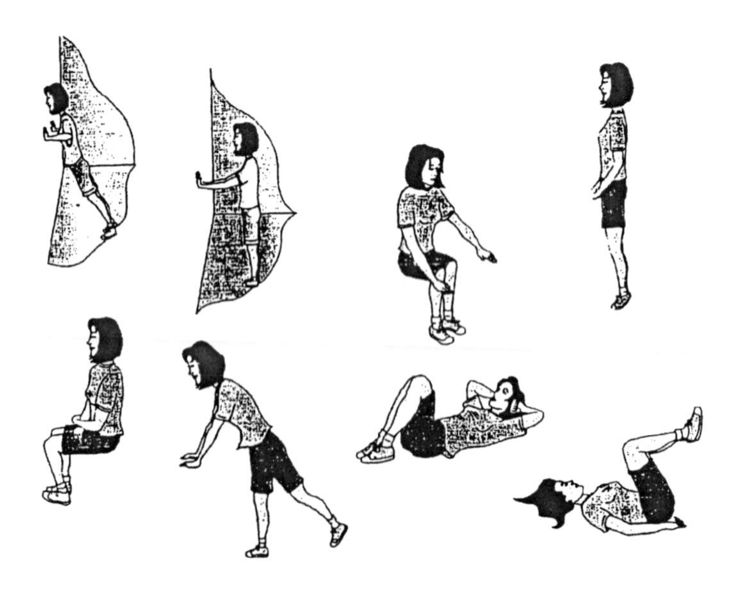

Another Green Level exercise is the Wall Pushaways for Triceps (arms) that is similar to the previous wall pushup, except for the hand position, which is side by side, instead of 6 - 8 inches apart. Lower Body exercises for the legs follow in three separate activities. "Calf Raises" is one of the Lower Body exercises. They are done by holding on to the back of a chair, raising your heels off the

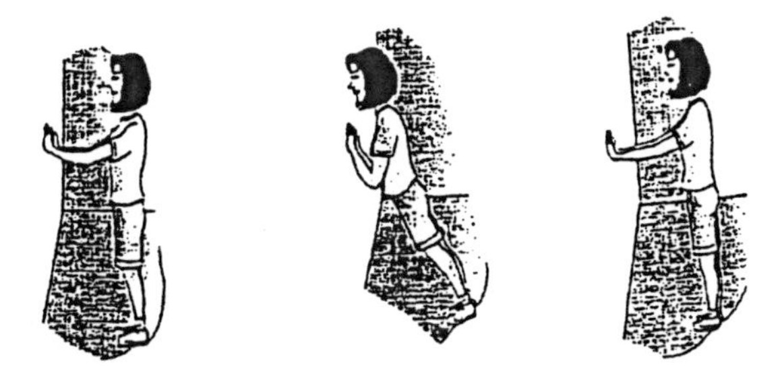

floor, with the weight on the balls of the feet, "tippy toes", exhaling, holding for a few seconds, and returning to the start position.

"The purpose of our butt muscles is to allow us to stand up, walk and climb stairs; and the purpose of the abdominal muscles is to assist in every activity we perform and help maintain a strong back and good posture," say the authors of *COMMERCIAL BREAK*. They have devised exercises to progressively strengthen and shape butt and abdominal muscles, while supporting the back of the head with the finger tips, but never pulling on the neck. Although it is normal for neck muscles to tire because the head weighs about eight pounds, neck muscles will gradually gain strength with the book's prescribed exercises. Green Level Butt and Gut exercises include "Butt Kickbacks", "Crunches", and " Roll-

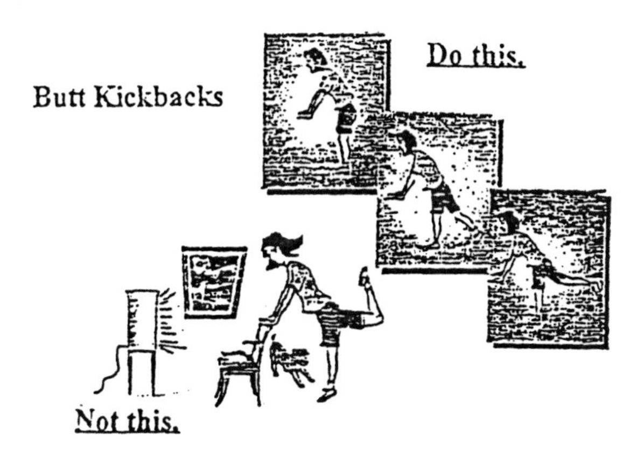

up Crunches", to be done at one commercial break.

Yellow-Level exercises are more challenging and should be tackled when you feel stronger, more flexible and steady on your feet. "Many women worry needlessly about becoming knuckle-dragging hulks by exercising their muscles," state the authors. They reassure readers that strong dense muscles will help reduce body fat and improve bone strength. Yellow Level exercises include Knee Pushups, Single Arm Triceps Pushups, Lunges, Calf Raises, Reclining Butt Crushers, Reversed Crunches, Side Crunches (for oblique or side muscles) and Bicycles.

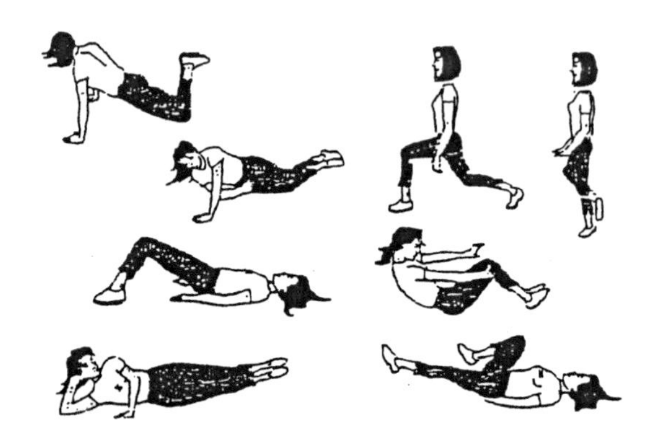

The book states that some parts of the body will improve quicker than others, so patience, persistence and consistency, as Cayce said, is necessary. Blue Level exercises are for those who mastered the Green and Yellow Levels. The goal of Blue Level is to perform the exercise for an entire commercial break. Blue Level exercises include Upper Body Elevated Pushups, Military Pushups, Elevated

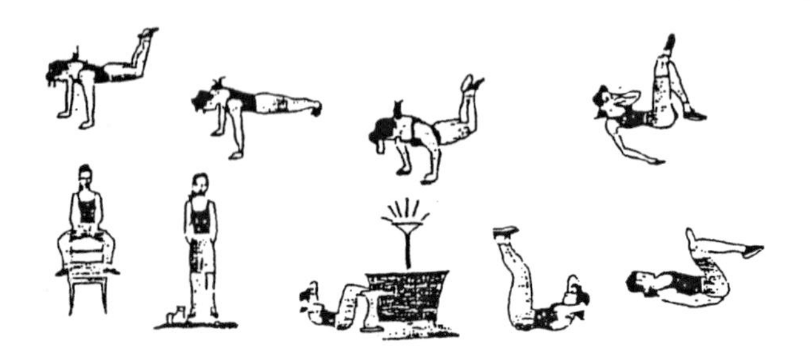

Triceps Pushups, Step-Ups, Plie' Squats, Calf Raises, Elevated Butt Crushers, Crunches, and Rollups.

Buch and Snider-Copley believe that people would strive to improve their odds against heart disease and other metabolic disorders associated with a sedentary lifestyle, if exercises were more accessible and "user friendly". Their Green, Yellow and Blue Level heart muscle exercises meet these requirements. They help prevent the heart and blood vessels from becoming brittle and/or clogged with "fatty 'goo" acquired from constantly eating high cholesterol foods. Odorless and waxy, cholesterol travels around the body via the blood stream. It cannot be tasted or seen, although it is in all animal food, and coconut and palm oils. We don't need cholesterol from food sources because the body produces enough and is the main source of cholesterol used to make essential substances such as cell walls and hormones.

Science has determined that a couch potato lifestyle, high in the consumption of animal products (meat, cheese, whole milk, cream) and low in fruits, vegetables, grains and beans, elevates blood cholesterol so that it cannot pass through the blood vessels. Instead, it will stick to the sides of blood vessels, building up like sludge on a kitchen pipe. Eating a variety of low fat, high fiber foods will result in HDLs (high density lipoproteins which are a combination of cholesterol, blood protein and fat in the blood) also known as good cholesterol. Bad cholesterol deposits fat sludge on the tissues and artery walls and is known as LDL (low density lipoprotein) and VLDL (very low density lipoproteins). HDL cholesterol is like little scouring pads that direct sludge in the blood to the liver for removal.

"Triglycerides" and "blood pressure" are other vocabulary discussed in *COMMERCIAL BREAK*. These are terms related to the heart and heart disease. Fats stored in the body are what triglycerides are about. The main job of triglycerides is to transport fat in the blood for use as energy. Fat not used, stores itself in the unlimited space of fat cells. These cells are known as adipose tissue. They are located in every part of the body: behind the kidneys for cushioning against bouncing or jarring; in a woman's breasts to protect her mammary glands; behind the skin to provide insulation and so forth. Fat is very necessary for optimum health, and is our primary energy source.

Blood pressure is the force flowing blood exerts against the walls of the arteries. Maximum pressure is exerted against the arterial walls when the heart contracts or "beats". A blood pressure reading of 120/80 is generally considered the norm, depending upon age, gender and family history. "If your blood pressure is high, it probably is due largely to dietary factors, sedentary lifestyle, smoking or genetic predisposition," say Buch and Snider-Copley. "Regular cardiovascular exercise is one way to control hypertension."

Scientists ascertain coronary risk by activity level, smoking, cholesterol, stress, and genetics. Buch and Snider-Copley's cardiovascular exercises stimulate the heart muscle and increase the breathing rate. They recommend proceeding slowly according to your exertion comfort level, which means paying attention to how you are feeling as you push harder in your workout. "If you are not comfortable with the exercise intensity, or you cannot say a few words without taking a breath, then slow down," state the authors. "Safe exercising is in the 50-80% range of what you perceive to be your maximum."

Green Level cardiovascular exercise is prefaced with several practical suggestions in *COMMERCIAL BREAK*:

1. replace soda, beer, or juice with water because water is the bodies preferred lubricant, while other beverages contain empty calories like sugar and caffeine which is a diuretic;

2. visit the 'john';

3. for every exercise level, be sure that you are wearing comfortable, supportive athletic shoes and clothing like a sweat suit and jog bra for the ladies;

4. have a towel handy;

5. for safety, clear the floor area of TV guides, remote control devices, cat toys, dog bones, sharp-edged tables and so forth;

6. for every exercise level, and during the course of the day when you are not consciously exercising, remember your posture, maintain proper alignment, tighten your abdominal muscles, relax your shoulders. It is also important to keep your head in a natural position comfortable between the shoulders, with eyes looking forward, and the chin parallel to the ground. A head out of alignment would have a dropped or raised chin which pinches the neck or spine, causing the shoulders to be tense or raised up toward the ears;

7. remember that your goal is to have fun!

8. after the exercise is finished, before flopping back on the couch, cool down by walking around for a minute or two to allow your heart rate to return to normal;

9. drink water after exercising. Normally, for intense workouts, a person would need about 4 ounces for every 15 - 20 minutes of exercise. Drinking an 8-ounce glass of water after the *COMMERCIAL BREAK* exercise program would be enough if one has been vigilant about water intake throughout the day.

Green Level cardiovascular exercise requires "Warm-Ups" during every commercial break for two hours of TV programming. "Warm-Ups" involve walking in place, swinging your arms in a controlled manner, elbows slightly bent and feet barely leaving the floor. "Stop exercising when your show resumes, drink water and relax," instruct Buch and Snider-Copley.

Yellow Level cardiovascular exercise indicates that your heart muscle is getting stronger. The "Ice Skater's Move", advised as a second exercise done during one commercial break, involves stepping from side-to-side like an ice skater, with right leg stepping to the right, then joined by the left leg; left leg steps back to the original position and is rejoined by the right leg. Arms swing naturally with the movement. The exercise is repeated as many times as you can for the duration of the commercial.

When you reach the Blue Level, "....you definitely 'have heart'," comment the authors. "Step-Ups", a Blue Level exercise, necessitates a step, bench, stair or footstool about 6 - 8 inches high that is secured to prevent slipping out from under you. Starting with your right leg, step on to the stair/bench/footstool with the entire foot, allowing the heel to strike first. The left foot then joins the right foot, followed by stepping back down to the floor, right foot first, followed by the left. The right foot leads for the rest of the commercial break. At the next commercial break, lead with the left foot, arms at sides, swinging normally. For more of a challenge, it is suggested that you lift arms overhead for the step up, bringing them back to shoulder level for the step down. The exercise is meant to be performed as a continuous pattern, without rest, with the goal being to perform the exercise at every commercial break for 2 hours of TV programming.

Chapter 9 in *COMMERCIAL BREAK*, is entitled: *The Food Factor*. It begins with an Old English proverb: "Don't dig your grave with your own knife and fork." The purpose of the chapter is to convey useful information, so readers can counter mindless eating prompted by poor choices and TV watching. These choices can pack on hundreds of unwanted calories and undermine good health. Some of the guiding facts and recommendations are:

1. Calories (defined as measures of energy) count, every single one of them, even "fat free" calories. 4 calories per gram are attributed to complex carbohydrates like fruits, vegetables, grains, beans/legumes, tubers, and simple carbohydrates like sugars, starches (potatoes) and processed grains and proteins

(meat, fish, dairy). Fats (butters, oils) are calculated at 9 calories per gram, and alcohol at 7 calories per gram. 3,500 calories = one pound of fat, but by reducing your daily intake of food by 250 calories, and doing a daily activity to burn 250 calories per day, you could probably lose about 1 pound per week.

2. It is never healthy to go below 1,200 calories per day, because the body needs at least 1,200 calories to maintain healthy bodily functions. Calories are energy. The organs, brain, liver, heart, muscles, cardiovascular system and other body systems require energy to run, much like a car needs gasoline in order to operate.

3. Eat breakfast, because your metabolism needs to be jump-started after sleeping 6 - 8 hours. For most people, nutritionists recommend that a healthy breakfast contain complex carbohydrates (fruit, grains, starches) and some protein (skim milk, yogurt, cottage cheese). High fiber cereals such as Shredded Wheat, Grape Nuts and Muselix are superior to cereals high in sugar and low in fiber. Soluble fiber, found in cellulose, gums, pectins, vegetables, fruits, whole grains, legumes, wheat bran, oat bran, nuts and seeds, helps retard the entry of glucose into the blood stream, absorbs cholesterol and gives the feeling of fullness when eating. Insoluble crude fiber comes from whole, unrefined grains, seeds and the woody parts of vegetables. The list of diseases that can be prevented or controlled by having the proper amount of dietary soluble and insoluble fiber is: heart disease, colon cancer, diverticulosis, diabetes, breast cancer, obesity, hemorrhoids, constipation and diarrhea.

4. Three ounces of protein, vegetables and grains are recommended for a healthy lunch. Dinner, "...should be the lightest meal of the day," say Buch and Snider-Copley. They suggest small snacks of about 250 calories, every 2-1/2 to 3 hours, like yogurt, veggies, fruit and crackers, so you don't go to bed hungry or feeling full. Government guidelines for good nutrition have changed from the four basic food groups: meat, dairy, fruit, vegetables and grains, to five basic food groups: vegetables, fruits, grains, meats and milk. The recommended caloric breakdown is: 55% carbohydrates (vegetables, fruit, rice, grains and complex starches), 20% protein (lean meat, poultry, fish and tofu) and 30% fats (oils, butter and margarine).

5. Portion size matters because the more you eat, the more calories you consume. It takes the body about 20 minutes to realize that it is full. Keeping portions sensibly sized keeps thousands of needless calories off your plate and body. A good measuring tool is your hand. Your palm = 3 ounces; your fist = 1 cup; a handful = 1 to 2 ounces of snack food; and your thumb = 1 ounce.

6. Keep precut vegetables and salad greens in the refrigerator. Take snacks like sliced oranges and apples, and a handful of almonds and walnuts to work. Have fresh fruit on the kitchen counter top, and place a bag of sweet baby carrots at eye level in the refrigerator. Stay well stocked in canned and frozen veggies and fruit. (According to the American Institute for Cancer Research (AICR), canned and frozen fruits and vegetables can provide even more nutrients then their fresh counterparts. New technologies, such as flash-freezing, trap nutrients and phytochemicals right after harvest when these foods are at their nutritional peak. Vitamin C and folate are extremely sensitive to changes in temperature, light and atmosphere; fresh fruits and vegetables stored at room temperature for two or three days can lose half their vitamin C, and as much as 70% of their folate. Make meat an added attraction, not the main event. Use a variety of fresh seasonings and spices. And when dining out, choose fresh veggies and fruit from the menu.

7. Eat one item per day that is red, orange, yellow, blue, green and purple so you meet the "five a day" fiber requirement.

8. Include a handful of nuts (almonds, pistachios, filberts, brazil nuts, peanuts and walnuts), and seeds (sesame, flax, pumpkin and sunflower) in your daily choice of food for essential fatty acids.

9. Drink plenty of water. An increase in fiber intake requires more water for better digestion. Water makes up about 60% of body weight, 70% of blood volume, and is part of the protein and glucose molecular structure. Water is an active participant in, and medium for, most body chemical reactions that keep you alive. "Drink water, or die," say Buch and Snider-Copley. The basic guidelines for water consumption and exercise are: 8 - 16 ounces of water 2 hours before exercise, and another 4 - 8 ounces prior to exercise. Drink 4 - 8 ounces of water during every 20 minutes of exercise at a commercial break. And drink 16 ounces of water for every pound of body weight you have lost. Increase water intake if you are fatigued, constipated, retain water or stuck on a weight loss plateau.

10. In 1984, the amount of sugar (cane, beet sugar, corn syrup and glucose) sold in the USA was about 125 pounds/year per person. By 1998, despite the increased use of artificial sweeteners, the amount of sugar consumed per person rose 25 % to 156 pounds/year per person. The increase is due to the fact that we are eating 1/3 more candy and 40% more sugary soft drinks than we did in 1984, with the amount of fat remaining status quo. Calorie intakes are up and so is obesity. Those who consume high sugar diets, honey, corn syrup and hybrid combinations like dextro-maltose, lose desire for essential fiber, calcium, iron,

magnesium, zinc, folate, niacin, riboflavin, and vitamins A, B-6, B-12, C, and E, and consume fewer fruits, veggies and dairy products. Sugar has also replaced many fat-free items, resulting in higher consumption of calories with fat-free foods because we erroneously believe that only fat has calories.

For those who are not permanently addicted to being couch potatoes, Buch and Snider-Copley recommend walking outdoors, which is an excellent exercise because walking is low impact and exercises the whole body. Cayce said: ***"After breakfast, work a while; after lunch, rest a while; after dinner, walk a mile."*** (3624-1). The authors, too, believe that a gentle walk after dinner improves digestion. But they say that walking with vigorous arm and leg movement after dinner could upset the digestive process. Buch and Snider-Copley believe that the best time for a vigorous walk is in the morning to foster better circulation, boost metabolism, encourage fat loss and reduce hypertension. They advise that a well constructed athletic shoe designed for walking or cross training is important for proper support. And a good running shoe works well for treks of longer duration or greater distances.

Swimming is another exercise highly recommended by Buch and Snider-Copley for most ages and physical conditions. Water exercise produces a general tonic effect on circulation, is non-impact, and even non-swimmers can get a great workout by just walking in the water. The authors recommend water aerobics classes as good exercise for everyone, including pregnant women, people with arthritis, osteoporosis and other disabling or painful afflictions, because water gives the body support and its resistance is soothing and invigorating.

"Little children, even infants, benefit from movement," say Buch and Snider-Copley. They believe that once a child is walking, they should be encouraged to participate in active play such as ball throwing, running, swimming, dancing, hopping, skipping and other fun activities involving large muscle motor skills for the legs, arms and torso. Older children can refine these skills by: jumping rope, hiking, biking, ball games, water games and sports, rollerblading, skiing, martial arts and other activities that build confidence, coordination, the ability to interact socially, and an appreciation of the body as an instrument of joy, fun and happiness. According to the authors, teenagers are inclined to be more competitive than younger children. They recommend team sports such as soccer, basketball, tennis, swimming, golf, track and field. "Recreational exercises that get the body moving, such as mountain biking, kayaking, surfing, and mountain/trail hiking, are an excellent way for families to enjoy healthy activities together," suggest Buch and Snider-Copley.

Seniors need to know, "...that it is never too late to get started on physical fitness," say the authors who cite research from Tufts University Human Nutrition Research Center, which indicates that two strength training sessions per week, for one year, halts or reverses the effects of aging, fragility, muscle weakness and arthritis, and other maladies associated with old age. Weight-bearing activities, like walking and strength training, improve bone density, making seniors less prone to bone fractures. A consistent program of strength training will raise the energy level as cardiovascular function improves, and, in turn, reduce stress and blood pressure.

"No matter what age you are, whether you are a couch potatoe or favor vigorous outdoor recreational exercise, a good base of muscle, flexibility and cardiovascular fitness is necessary for wellness and enjoyment of life," say Buch and Snider-Copley. They recommend reading *Getting Old Is Not For Sissies: Portraits Of Senior Athletes,* by Etta Clark, a book about men and women, age 60 to 100 who enjoy yoga, judo, surfing, skiing, swimming, biking and other sports and exercises. "At all ages life is meant to be enjoyed with activities that encourage fitness," say the authors.

And couch potatoes, too, like my friend Annie used to be, are changing their lives for the better, by "MOVING", diet and the easy exercises in *COMMERCIAL BREAK*, without ever interrupting their favorite TV shows.

"Now that's entertainment!" Annie says.

....

Linda Buch and Seth Anne Snider-Copley can be contacted at:

Balance/Fitness Books, LLC
22 South Nome Street, # E
Aurora, Colorado 80012
Phone: 303-363-9057
Email: LJBalance@aol.com

....

COMMERCIAL BREAK: The Complete Couch Potato's Guide to Fitness, was recently acquired by Prima Publishing, a Crown/Random House Subsidiary. The new edition, published by Prima, is titled:

THE COMMERCIAL BREAK WORKOUT

For Information About Alternative Health Care Techniques To Improve Posture/Balance and Other Structural Problems, Contact:

1) Yoga (check your Yellow Pages and local rec center's for Yoga classes)

2) Pilates 505 - 988 - 1990

3) Swiss Ball Dynamics 800 - 752 - 2255

4) Alexander Technique 800 - 473 - 0620

5) Feldenkrais Method 800 - 775 - 2118

....

RECOMMENDED READING

THE ULTIMATE FIT OR FAT
Covert Bailey
Houghton Mifflin, 2000

SMART EXERCISE
Covert Bailey
Houghton Mifflin, 1994

STRETCH FOR HEALTH:
The Edgar Cayce Way To Energize
Edgar Cayce Foundation, 1990
(Videotape)
Available through the A.R.E. Bookstore

1-800-723-1112

6

"GRANDMOTHER OF HOLISTIC HEALTH"
Rev. Hanna Kroeger

....

Women were always healers -
naturally born healers.
They hold the crying child and
soothe their needs (psychiatrist).
They dig out the thorn from the finger (surgeon).
They ease the fever (internist).
They dress the sores and bathe their
beloved ones in herbs (herbalist).
They dry the tears (minister).

Hanna Kroeger
From: *GOD HELPS THOSE*
WHO HELP THEMSELVES

....

(Use) those things that are as medicines,
or as of nature's storehouse,
or of that known rather as the naturopath -
in the use to be sure of herbs.

EDGAR CAYCE
Reading 1221-1

....

The late **Rev. Hanna Kroeger**, dubbed "Grandmother of Holistic Health", was known and respected among health care professionals, as a master herbalist and natural healer. She was the daughter of German Christian missionaries. Rev. Kroeger studied nursing at the University of Freiberg, Germany. While working at a Dresden hospital that used natural healing methods, she learned how herbs could cure illness. Her life was devoted to helping people regain good health with herbs, diet, homeopathic medicine, vitamins, magnets, physical alignment, Christ healing, massage, reflexology, aura balancing, dowsing, stones and crystals, flower essences, color, mind power, healing from a distance, residue healing and other unusual vibrational and natural healing techniques. She authored more than twenty books on old and new home remedies, self-healing techniques, special diets, physical, mental and spiritual causes of illness, herbal and vitamin references and cookbooks.

....

Wholistic health represents an attitude toward well-being which
recognizes that we are not just a collection of mechanical parts,
but an integrated system which is physical, mental, social and spiritual.

Hanna Kroeger
From: *GOD HELPS THOSE WHO HELP THEMSELVES*

....

The human body is made up electronic vibrations,
with each atom and every element of the body,
each organ and organism having its electronic
unit of vibration necessary for the sustenance of,
and equilibrium in that particular organism.

Thomas J. Sugrue
From: *THERE IS A RIVER*

....

REV. HANNA KROEGER'S CHAPEL OF MIRACLES

It is early Sunday morning in Boulder, Colorado. I am driving, with my friend Karen, along Valmont Road, deep into the countryside. We are going to a healing service at Rev. Hanna Kroeger's Chapel of Miracles. Karen is suffering from bouts of extreme fatigue, frequent headaches and indigestion. She says she has been diagnosed with Candida Albicans, an abnormally high fungus in the intestinal tract. Conventional medicine has failed her and she is hoping that Hanna Kroeger, the master herbalist, natural healer, can help her.

We drive past cows and horses grazing on the lush Colorado countryside. "There it is!" Karen announces pointing to a blue triangular sign peeking out from the foliage. It says "Chapel of Miracles" in large, white hand-printed letters. An illustration of a flying white dove is centered above the lettering. I make a sharp left turn at the sign and drive along a dirt road thick with autumn foliage and wild purple and white flowers. At the end of the road another sign points to "Hanna's Retreat". I drive through an open chicken wire fence, down the dirt road, to a humble, rambling old farm house. It is surrounded by a majestic view of the snow-capped Rocky Mountains. I park near a church bell mounted on a wooden pole. We walk past a stone statue of the Virgin Mary surrounded by ceramic angels and pots of pastel flowers. On the west end of Hanna's "L" shaped house is a hand-painted sign that says: *"Lord, there is no one besides thee to help." 2 Chronicles, 14:11.* Beneath the sign is a small stone statue of Saint Francis.

A large wooden crucifix adorns the facade of the entrance to the house. I hesitate before knocking, because we are early and no one has arrived yet for the 9:30 a.m. service. Hanna Kroeger, a poised, handsome, fair-skinned woman in her 80s, opens the door. She is trim and tiny, evoking a magical presence of combined innocence and worldly sophistication. I sense a youthful energy and good humor about her. Hanna's face is lined with fine wrinkles and laugh lines defining the corners of her mouth. A warm, friendly smile reveals teeth graying with age. Her penetrating blue-gray eyes shine with intelligence. Hanna is wearing a calf length, navy-blue, long-sleeved dress, and a matching sash wrapped around her softly swept up gray hair. Pinned to the left corner of her white crocheted collar is a small gold cross shining with reflected sunlight. She wears dark stockings and sensible black laced shoes. And in her right hand, a metal pendulum dangles from a chain.

"Good morning! What can I do for you?" she asks cheerfully in a German accent.

"I wonder if you can help me, I have Candida," Karen answers.

She invites us into her comfortable country kitchen. A pleasant aroma of sponge cake fills the room. She is baking for the church congregation. Karen tells Hanna about her symptoms while Hanna studies Karen's aura intently. The aura is an energy invisible to the naked eye, that emanates from each organ of the body, but can be seen by "sensitives". Hanna touches Karen beneath her arm and behind her ear lobes. "You have swollen lymph glands," she remarks. Then she presses on Karen's palm and asks if it hurts. Karen nods yes. Fascinated, I watch Hanna's steady hand pass the gyrating pendulum over Karen's body. The pendulum twirls in a circle on some parts of Karen's body and swings back and forth on other parts of her anatomy.

"You don't have Candida," Hanna concludes. "You have Epstein-Barr Syndrome which resembles Mononucleosis. Both diseases are viruses in the lymphatic system. They can be taken care of with herbs, lettuce leaves and homeopathic medicine." She recommends that Karen drink one-quart of red raspberry tea daily, apply raw tomato poultices to her neck for the swelling induced by Epstein-Barr Syndrome, and to take an herbal formula of raspberry leaves, lettuce, eucalyptus, club moss, tarragon, condurango bark and jasmine. Hanna says, "These ingredients are obtained from our Lords drugstore, and are available at health food stores." Hanna's Herb Shop, located a few blocks from her home, carries herbs and homeopathic medicine to treat Epstein-Barr Virus.

"How does the pendulum work?" I ask. Hanna explains that life is vibrational energy, and the pendulum operates on this manifestation. It gyrates over the body because electromagnetic frequencies are transmitted by healthy organs. The pendulum does not gyrate over ailing parts of the body. Instead, it swings back and forth when no vibrational electro magnetic energy is transmitted.

The diagnosis is that Karen has roundworms in her intestines. "For the next two days, eat as much garlic as you can stand. Then take a laxative," Hanna tells her. "This may be unpleasant - sit in a milk bath covering the rectal area for one hour. The worms will smell the milk and crawl out." She also recommends an herbal combination of black walnut leaves, wormwood, guassia, cloves and male fern.

Hanna believes that everyone has worms and/or parasites. She tells us that we can often be infected from our pet cats and dogs. According to Hanna, invasion of one or more of over 120 parasites and worms, can, and do, invade the body. This can occur when the liver cannot neutralize chemicals, metals and environmental poisons. It also can happen when the colon is toxic and the body has an alkaline medium. Hanna warns that worms and parasites take nutrients from the blood and leave their poisonous wastes. "They disturb the balance of the body system and can cause mineral imbalance, loss of hair, loss of sleep, headaches, thyroid imbalances, intestinal gas, blood in the stool, chronic prostatis, allergies, eczema, pain all over the body, arthritis and high blood sugar," she tells us.

"Do I have parasites?" I ask with concern. "Is that why I have been suffering from headaches?"

Hanna examines me with the gyrating pendulum. "Take equal parts of the natural oils of sassafras, wintergreen and spruce to rid your body of blood parasites. Once they are gone, your headaches will disappear," she informs me. "Also, rub 4 drops of the mixture on the soles of your feet, three times a day." Hanna tells me that pumpkin seeds are an excellent anti-parasitic, and that two-teaspoons of apple cider vinegar, taken every day in an 8 oz. glass of water, will prevent parasites from entering my body.

People are beginning to arrive. Hanna excuses herself, checks the oven and removes the baking pans. While she is arranging the cake on platters, a well-groomed, middle-aged woman in a business suit enters the room. She has brought her aunt for a healing. We strike up a conversation. The woman says that she went from doctor to doctor trying to get her heart rhythms back to normal. She had no success until Hanna prescribed herbs and homeopathic medicines. Her heart is now beating normally, and she wants Hanna to help her aunt with a similar problem.

One of Hanna's assistants is ringing the church bell. Many vehicles, from motorcycles to Mercedes, are parked outside the house. People of all ages, cultures and walks of life are assembling for the service. We follow Hanna to the upstairs chapel in her house. Over one hundred people are seated on the cushioned pews.

Religious art decorates the walls of the simple white-washed sanctuary. Lantern-type lights fastened to chains hang from exposed ceiling beams. Adorning the pulpit are dozens of red and white lit candles, a cross covered with white lilies, ceramic angels and a statue of the Virgin Mary. The chapel windows face a postcard-pretty view of the rugged snow-capped mountains.

Hanna steps up on the platform and speaks into a microphone, "Does anyone have special hymn preferences today?" Someone answers, *Holy, Holy, Holy.* The man seated at the organ begins to play, as people open their book of hymns and sing in unison. After the singing, Hanna begins the sermon. She tells us that when she first came to this country and applied for citizenship, the judge at the ceremony said, "You came to America not to take a loan, but to contribute your skills and special gifts so we all thrive." Hanna confides to the congregation that she never forgot those words, and has happily lived accordingly. "We must pray for freedom and never take it for granted," she says.

The right way to pray, so God can hear you, is demonstrated by Hanna. She holds her hands facing upward, tent style, palms apart, with the tips of her fingers touching. "When the hands are in this position, they transmit energy," she explains. "The energy is cut off when you hold your palms together." She demonstrates the concept with the pendulum, on a man seated in the front row. He is holding his hands in the prayer position, palms apart. When Hanna steps many feet away from the man, her pendulum continues to gyrate. But when the man holds his palms together in the prayer position, her pendulum stops gyrating, and swings back and forth, because the energy is cut off.

"Never be afraid to speak up for freedom. You'd be amazed at the power one person has to overcome injustice," Hanna says. She tells us that recently she was in an airport on her way to do a lecture in another State. Enroute to the departure gate she witnessed a man abusing a woman. "People walked by doing nothing to aid the woman," she relates. "I never pass by an injustice and say nothing." Although she was late, and thought she might miss her plane, she confronted the man, told him his behavior was intolerable and smacked him. "I did not smack him hard and I did not miss my plane," she informs a chuckling audience. "But I did stop the man from abusing the woman for a moment."

Hanna picks up a large pile of letters and shows them to us. "People have written to me asking for help for many physical, mental and spiritual problems," she informs the congregation. She places the correspondence in the center of the floor and asks us to help expel the bad forces invading these lives by saying, "Be bound!" We repeat the words three times in unison. Then Hanna requests that we join her in singing *How Great Thou Art*.

Services end with *The Lord's Prayer*. The congregation rises and goes downstairs to another chapel jammed with people. They are waiting for diagnosis and recommended treatment from Hanna and her assistants. There is no fee for the healing, although I notice several people leaving donations in a box near the door. I watch as Hanna efficiently tends to each person with a pleasant, but no-nonsense approach. As Karen and I leave, we hear Hanna saying to a woman, "The crease in your ear lobe indicates that you have heart problems."

We head down Valmont Road to Hanna's Herbal Shop. Flyers in the shop explain that Hanna arrived in America from Germany in the early 1950s. Disappointed by the lack of nutritious food, she bought bulk whole grains, made fresh carrot juice, and combined subtle and unique combinations of herbs to improve the health of friends and family. This grew into one of the first health food stores in the United States. In 1978 she started Kroeger Herb Products to keep up with the growing demand for her formulas.

The store is very interesting. Clerks are friendly, informative and helpful. There is a table with fresh orange juice and an assortment of delicious looking muffins. "Please help yourself," the clerk tells us. Shelves of herbal and homeopathic remedies line the walls. Natural cosmetics, toothpaste with no aluminum in it, therapeutic magnets and other unusual healing devices are displayed on draped tables with explanatory literature.

I decide to buy a Soma Board designed by Hanna. It is a small box, approximately 4" x 6" x 1", with a washable top, containing a unique blend of minerals and herbs. The brochure explains that the Soma Board will bring healthful vibrations to vegetables, fruit, water, milk, juice and bread that is placed on top of it. It will also improve the taste of food. The Soma Board operates on the principle of pyramid energy, neutralizing metals and chemicals by ionizing them so they are harmless.

Karen buys a Water Revitalizer Disc. The directions say to place a glass of fluid on the magnetized disc to draw magnetism into the fluid. This is supposed to restore natural magnetic energy and balance to your body's magnetic field. Physical, mental, emotional, and magnetic balance prevents us from becoming ill, or staying ill for long.

At the rear of the shop is a display of books on health and healing written by Hanna and other authors. I thumb through Hanna's *New Book On Healing*, and read her recommendation on treatment for cataracts. It says, "Take fresh coconut juice, and with an eye dropper, apply as much as the eye can hold. Apply hot cloths for about 10 minutes while lying down. Several treatments are needed." The book is an anthology of tried and tested, ancient and up-to-date, common sense, natural healing remedies for body, mind and spirit. I buy it.

The clerk finds kits with the herbal and homeopathic medicines that Hanna has recommended for Karen and me. "If these remedies do not work, can I return them?" Karen asks. "Yes," answers the clerk. Karen says she wants to go to her medical doctor for a second opinion before she takes the herbs and homeopathic medicine. Since the experience has been so unusual, I decide to do the same.

On Monday we go to our respective physicians for tests; they confirm Hanna's diagnosis. We follow her treatment plan with excellent results. Karen no longer has Epstein-Barr Virus Syndrome or roundworms. And I have rid myself of pinworms and headaches. We are amazed at Hanna's accurate findings, and marvel at her healing skills. Karen and I agree, Hanna is an extraordinary woman! Yet she does not claim to have any outstanding gifts, only that they are from a higher power. At the core of her unique healing style is her devout belief that God can heal any ailment at any time. We look forward to attending another Sunday service and visiting the unforgettable Hanna Kroeger again.

....

May the angels of love heal you.

Hanna Kroeger

....

On May 7, 1998, Rev. Hanna Kroeger passed away. Her family and the practitioners trained by Hanna Kroeger carry on her work. Services are held, as usual, on Sunday mornings at 9:30 a.m., followed by healings with Rev. Kroeger's proteges at the Chapel of Miracles.

PSYCHOMETRIC AURIC ENERGY MEASUREMENT

Auric energies of the body can be measured psychometrically using a saliva sample. From these readings recommendations will be made by health care practitioners at the Chapel of Miracles to help increase the aura vitality of your organs. This is a spiritual reading not intended to replace or discourage a regular visit to your physician.

1. Wet a small piece of cotton early in the morning with the saliva of the person for whom you want the reading. A nickel size dab is fine.

2. Wrap the cotton ball in a clear plastic bag. Be sure to seal it tightly. Write a brief paragraph that includes your name, return address, age, major complaints, any available medical diagnosis and what you have done about your condition (s).

3. A donation of $20 is requested. Make check or money order payable to: The Chapel of Miracles. (Credit cards not accepted)

4. Please include two self-addressed stamped envelopes and mail them to:

Chapel of Miracles
7075 Valmont Road
Boulder, CO 80301

...there IS that principle in every herb,
yes in every element, that is creative within itself that
gives that inclination for HEALING to a physical body...

EDGAR CAYCE
Reading 1458-1

RECOMMENDED BOOKS

Books By Rev. Hanna Kroeger
(Hanna Kroeger Publications)

HOW TO COUNTERACT ENVIRONMENTAL POISONS, 1990

PARASITES: THE ENEMY WITHIN, 1991

OLD-TIME REMEDIES FOR MODERN AILMENTS, 1971

NEW BOOK ON HEALING, 1996

GOOD HEALTH THROUGH SPECIAL DIETS, 1981

GOD HELPS THOSE WHO HELP THEMSELVES, 1984

AGELESS REMEDIES FROM MOTHER'S KITCHEN, 1981

For one year I worked on the phenomenon of the pendulum. I took my wedding ring and hung it on a thread, dangling it over my hands, my knees, my food, and sure enough, slowly the ring started gyrating. I steadied myself in every way possible but the ring kept moving.

Hanna Kroeger
From: *GOD HELPS THOSE WHO HELP THEMSELVES*

....

7

SIMPLE HEALING TECHNIQUES FOR IMPROVING VISION

Interview With Joy Thompson, Vision Educator

....

[Cayce's] general recommendations [for eye care] include maintaining the cervical and upper dorsal vertebrae in proper alignment and consuming raw vegetables (especially carrots) with gelatin and citrus fruits as part of the diet. To specifically help maintain visual acuity, the readings recommend the daily use of the head-and-neck exercises...

ERIC MEIN, M.D.
From: *Keys To Health*

JoyThompson is a vision educator. She began studying techniques for vision correction in 1994 as a way to find a better answer to corrective lenses. In an article that she wrote for *Venture Inward*, the A.R.E.'s monthly magazine, Thompson told readers that her doctors prescribed eyeglasses as the only choice for Gwen, her nearsighted 11-year old daughter. Their prognosis for Gwen's visual improvement was bleak. And their forecast was equally disheartening for Thompson's recovery from difficulty in reading fine print. They referred to her eyesight as "middle-aged", farsighted, blurred vision, or "presbyopia". Doctors even predicted further deterioration of Thompson's vision as she aged, with reading glasses as her single option. Unlike her doctors, she believed that deficient vision was largely due to factors which were correctable. Thompson asked herself why the eyes could not heal if the rest of the body was capable of doing so. She observed that "corrective" lenses, did not actually correct the problem, but were much like drug therapy, which treated the symptom, not the root cause of the problem. This lead Thompson to begin her search for alternative answers to eye care.

In the case of Gwen, her nearsighted vision coincided with the onset of puberty and a great deal of stress at school. Gwen was becoming more introverted and withdrawn, using her eyes in a stressful, imbalanced way. She spent many hours in "nearsighted" activities: reading, watching TV, playing computer games, staying indoors out of the sunshine, and not involving her eyes in distance viewing. Using her intuition, Thompson knew that "outer vision" and "inner vision" were synonymous with "sight" and "insight". She also knew that fear and stress were causing eye problems for her and her daughter.

Thompson began studies on holistic eye treatment. She attended workshops lead by alternative eye care specialist Elizabeth Abraham, Director of Toronto's Vision Improvement Center. Classes focused on the work of optometrist William Bates, author of the 1940 revolutionary book *Better Eyesight Without Glasses*. Bates' work confirmed Thompson's belief that negative emotions, stress, exhaustion and poor diet were usually primary factors playing a crucial role in undermining vision. Thompson and her daughter practiced the holistic philosophy and program of easy eye exercises prescribed by Bates. Done for a few moments each day, their sight improved considerably. It was this success that motivated Thompson to become a vision educator.

Gwen's vision improvement program consisted of exercises and practices designed to relax the eyes, since eye tension is the primary cause of myopia (nearsightedness). Taking regular breaks from near-distance activities included: resting her eyes by looking far into the distance, massaging acupressure points on her eyes, palming (resting the closed eyes under cupped palms) and stimulating her eyes with full spectrum light. She also began a study of Tai Chi, a practice which helps move energy in the body and encourages a deep relaxed state of mind and body. Gwen avoided carbonated drinks and excessive sweets and fats. She followed a light vegetarian diet, eating organic fruit and vegetables, whenever possible.

Thompson continued training with Dr. Robert-Michael Kaplan of Sechelt, British Columbia. He is the author of *The Power Behind Your Eyes* and *Seeing Without Glasses*. After 11 days of concentrated work on her eyes with Kaplan, Thompson's "middle-age" farsightedness was repaired. Her fear of facing the future disappeared, too, and she was able to create a new positive vision for her life. Upon conclusion of her studies, she began her career as a vision coach. Thompson is dedicated to educating people of all ages, on the art and science of naturally improving vision. She has had many successes, including her daughter Gwen's reduced lens prescription, and freeing her clients from progressive dependency on eyeglasses.

INTERVIEW WITH
JOY THOMPSON, VISION COACH

BETTE: I understand that eyes are the body's most highly developed sensory organ, housing 70% of its sense receptors. What portion of the brain is dedicated to the function of eyesight?

JOY: The posterior third of the brain is used for vision and houses the memory bank which is attributed to much of our intelligence. Every second, two million messages are sent to the brain through the eyes.

BETTE: That's a pretty formidable task considering that the eyes represent only 2% of our body weight.

JOY: But the eyes require 25% of our nutritional intake and use one-third as much oxygen as the heart. They need about 20 times as much vitamin C as the joints involved in the movement of extremities.

BETTE: How do you determine the most beneficial treatment for a client's eye condition?

JOY: Initially, I test a client's eyes for visual clarity at a distance and at the near point. Then I examine how the eyes work individually and together as a team. My program for optimum eye care improvement is based on the results of these tests and the client's resolution to make changes in lifestyle. This includes attitude, stress, diet and a commitment to follow through with implementing eye exercises. There are no "quick fixes", so patience is required while waiting for vision improvements to occur.

BETTE: Do you implement a support system to help your clients stick to the program?

JOY: I extend a great deal of support, by being available via telephone or email, at all times. The first month of treatment seems to be critical for people. I have hosted support groups in the past and am currently forming another one. As the client's visual system begins to respond, their program is modified and new goals are set.

BETTE: Would you give an example of a program for someone with severe myopia (near-sightedness)?

JOY: I would suggest to the client that for the first month they work daily to stimulate the eyes with sunlight, practice massaging the eyes and "palming" them regularly to relax the visual system. Stimulating the eyes with sunlight is called "sunning" by Dr. William Bates. Sunning is to the eyes what the sauna/cold shower routine is for the body. When we are in a sauna, tiny capillaries enlarge in response to the heat and then shrink suddenly in a cold shower. This is a workout for the vascular system. Similarly, with sunning, we bathe the eyes in bright sunlight by turning the closed eyelids toward the sun while rotating the head slowly, side to side. This is followed by relaxing the visual system in darkness through "palming", a method for eye wellness that generally improves and maintains vision. Palming was practiced by yoga masters as early as 500 BC.

BETTE: How is palming done?

JOY: Rub the palms of the hands together to generate warmth and energy. Then place the cupped palms over closed eyelids, so there is an energetic pocket of warm air over the eyes, which draws in energy from the palms. Visualizing something black affects muscle relaxation during this process, which can be done for any length of time. The rods and cones in the eyes close tightly when stimulated by bright sun, and then open wide in the darkness. When the hands are removed from the eyes, the lids should remain closed for a minute so the eyes can adjust to the light before opening them. For the eyes to work more efficiently in using or blocking light, palming should be repeated twice daily. Palming also improves night blindness and light sensitivity. The exercise is like a mini-vacation for the eyes and generally improves and maintains vision.

BETTE: I understand that eye massage is also beneficial for eye health. How do you do this?

JOY: Gently massaging the eyes is very helpful for arousing circulation. It encourages the eye muscle to relax by stimulating acupressure points above and below the corners, and above and below the center of the eyes. Massage should be done delicately between the eyebrow bone and eyeball. That's the hollow area where the eye muscle lives. Also massage the tear ducts which are the bumps in the corners of the eyes. This is done with a gentle pressure of the thumb and forefinger followed by palming.

BETTE: How long would it take for a severely myopic patient to see some improvement?

JOY: Normally it would take about a month for improvement to surface. The next step would be to wear a patch, for several hours each day, over the stronger eye, if this was a factor, as it often is. Patching would stimulate the weaker eye and improvement in eyesight would result. The third step might be eye muscle exercises to get both eyes working together as a team. Creating new visual habits supports healing the eyes for clearer vision. Frequently there is also positive emotional transformation which results from vision clearing.

BETTE: Does palming improve focus of farsightedness?

JOY: Yes, indirectly. The eyes respond quickly to palming. And it benefits clarity of focus once the eyes relax and the eye muscles flex tighter. This is done by shifting focus on various distances far away and then as close up as placing your thumb in front of your nose so your eyes cross.

BETTE: Are there other exercises to improve nearsightedness and farsightedness?

JOY: There are dozens. A very simple maintenance exercise for vision fitness is one I call "shifting". Start by looking into the far distance letting your eyes focus on something. In my case, here in Vancouver, I would gaze at the mountains. Then look at something closer, like a tree across the street. Then shift closer, perhaps to the fence in your yard. And finally, focus on your thumb which you hold in front of your nose. Repeat the sequence several times - mountains, tree, fence, thumb - and your eyes will get a focusing workout. Another basic exercise is to follow your thumb, or a pencil, with your vision as you move it towards your nose so your eyes cross. This encourages the eye muscles to work together to keep a single image. Practice this several times a day to keep your near focus sharp. And, yes, crossing your eyes is good for you!

BETTE: Do some people heal their eyes faster than others?

JOY: I have had clients who made incredible progress. Several have changed their nearsighted prescriptions within a few weeks of eye exercises. That is because the eyeglasses they had to begin with were too strong. Two of my clients even healed their astigmatism, (a distortion of one plane of view which can affect one or both eyes). Generally, an astigmatism is considered untreatable except by using special prescriptive lenses. But these astigmatic cases were gone within one year of adopting a natural eye care program.

BETTE: Are there any other personal practices that aid in maintaining and improving eyesight?

JOY: I teach Yoga stretches and movements to relax the neck and shoulders and keep energy moving. Yoga is effective in improvement and maintenance of good vision. Acupressure treatments are another effectual means for releasing tight muscles and moving blocked energy. And Tai Chi or Chi Gung are also very helpful in keeping energy moving through the body into the eyes, encouraging a more relaxed physical state. Meditation and visualization are profound as well. A general exercise program of swimming, cycling, and/or running is also beneficial. Sports which encourage distance focus, like the eye following a ball into the distance, are tennis, basketball or hockey. These games contribute to strengthening vision and play a part in curing myopia. Near vision activities such as reading, sewing and woodworking require good lighting, taking regular breaks and compensating with far-distance viewing to alleviate farsightedness (presbyopia). And of course, a healthy diet is essential for general well-being which includes good eye health.

BETTE: What do you consider a healthy diet?

JOY: Basically, a vegetarian diet. Whenever possible, use organic foods which are higher in nutritive value than non-organic foods. Raw and lightly cooked vegetables are an important source of vitamins and minerals necessary for eye health. A vegetarian diet is the kindest way to treat the body along with supplementation of trace minerals found in sea vegetables like algae, nori, dulse and spirolina. Herbal teas, especially peppermint tea, are also good for the eyes. Caffeine, carbonated drinks, alcohol, red meat and refined sugar should be kept to a minimum. Potato chips, fatty meats, cheeses and butter should be eliminated or drastically reduced from most diets. We need fat in our diet, but in much lower quantities than most people think. Drinking lots of spring water is also beneficial for the whole body.

BETTE: Which vitamins and/or minerals do you recommend?

JOY: Vitamin A is good for impaired night vision. It is found in liver, parsley, carrots, butter, egg yolk and green leafy vegetables. I also recommend: B1, B2, B12, C and E. B1 is in beans, nuts, wheat germ, potatoes, yeast and broccoli. B2 is in vegetables, fowl, milk, yeast, soybeans and eggs. B12, important for alleviating light sensitivity, is in fish, eggs and yeast. C is found in citrus fruit, green leafy vegetables and parsley. E, which is beneficial for blood circulation to the eyes, is in cold pressed vegetable oils, seeds and nuts, wheat germ and green leafy vegetables.

BETTE: Are there other health food supplements that you suggest?

JOY: It depends upon the circumstances. One client came to me with eye pressures at the dangerous level of 22 and 20. He decided not to take his doctor's prescribed eye drops because he knew he could become dependent upon them. Instead, he followed a natural eye care regimen. This involved an oral supplement of 120 mg. of gingko daily, palming often during the day, and eye patching to strengthen the weaker eye so it worked as a team with the stronger eye. He also did the head and neck exercises recommended over 300 times in Cayce's readings. And he continued with his personal Tai Chi practice. Within six months his eye pressures reduced to 15 and 14, which is slightly lower than normal.

BETTE: When and how are Cayce's head and neck exercises done?

JOY: They are done twice a day, as Cayce suggested - in the morning standing up, and in the evening sitting down. The exercises consist of slowly and gently bending the head 3 times to the right, 3 times to the left, forward 3 times, backward 3 times, 3 times full circle clockwise, and 3 times full circle counter clockwise. Head and neck exercises increase circulation through the carotid artery in the side of the neck, augmenting the energy flow through the shoulders and neck to the face and ears. It is very important that this exercise be done slowly and mindfully, because it is powerful enough to cause headaches or dizziness if done quickly. Many health problems are rooted in withdrawal of energy or too much build up of energy. Done properly, head and neck exercises can stabilize or activate energy, stimulate and heal the eyes and encourage communication between the body and mind. In our culture, we tend to "live in our heads". The head and neck exercises can get the body in touch with the brain.

BETTE: Is there a treatment to correct color blindness?

JOY: I am not aware of any cases in which color blindness has been reversed. However, a client of mine told me that his teachers in grade school assumed he was a slow learner, when in reality the problem was that he was color blind. After diagnosing his condition, they drilled him on how to distinguish colors through intensity and vibration, which is how looking at the color affects the observer. As a result of this early training, he can now recognize certain shades of a color, even though he sees only in black, white and gray.

BETTE: Can night blindness be improved?

JOY: I believe impaired night vision is caused by lack of light stimulation, resulting in a weak visual system. A diet high in vitamins, especially vitamin A, is very beneficial for improving night blindness. Using light stimulation or "sunning", can improve night blindness and light sensitivity. Also, the herb bilberry has proven to be effective for impaired night vision. British pilots took bilberry during the war to keep their night vision sharp.

BETTE: Do you have any remedies for conjunctivitis?

JOY: Whenever I see a suffix with "itis", I assume that stress, strain and anger are rooted in the ailment. This certainly has been my experience with conjunctivitis. People who continually drive themselves to accomplish and achieve goals often experience eyestrain. When left untreated, eyestrain results in conjunctivitis infection. The remedy that I prescribe for this condition is relaxation, stress management and attention to diet. People should be careful to minimize, or better yet, eliminate fast foods with high sodium content. The hard-driving, type A personality that often develops conjunctivitis is also the type who typically doesn't eat well. If the client uses a computer, I educate him/her about prevention of computer eyestrain. I believe that eyestrain can be a direct cause of the weakened visual system which contracts the conjunctivitis infection. A cool cloth or eye pillow can help ease the condition. But if it persists, a doctor's prescription for drops will be necessary. However, the condition will return for certain people if they don't make changes in how they treat themselves and their eyes.

BETTE: How can computer eye abuse be prevented?

JOY: Never work at the computer more than 25 minutes without taking a break. The break can be as short as two minutes, but it benefits the eyes.

BETTE: What other factors contribute to the mistreatment of the eyes?

JOY: Our eyes are meant to be stimulated by bright sunlight every day, and to rest in deep darkness at night. Many unhealthy modern habits have increased vision problems. General mistreatment of our eyes includes: the use of artificial light, long eye straining work days for 11 months, before taking a vacation, excessive TV watching, and eye overuse for lengthy reading, studying, driving and computer work, with no regard to balancing near and far distance seeing. The stress of modern living, and falling asleep nightly with tense eyes, which is responsible for starting a new day with tense eyes, also largely contributes to abuse of the eyes.

BETTE: How can bad reading habits be mended?

JOY: Place a bookmark, about 20 minutes reading time, ahead in the book. Stop at that point, take a break, breathe deeply, relax, stretch, blink, look away into the distance, palm and then resume reading. This ritual can take 3 minutes or less.

By evening the eyes are tired or strained from being used during the day. Whenever possible, read earlier in the day. Reading material should be held about 14 inches away from the eyes, with the eyes at ease looking downward. One of the worst reading habits of all is reading in bed, because posture is usually poor. The best way to read is sitting with the back comfortably straight on a chair or sofa, under good lighting. Natural, full-spectrum lighting is readily available these days and should be utilized to read with relaxed eyes. This is a very important skill, because reading with tense eyes creates even more tension, causing increased eye problems. The cycle of eye mistreatment must be broken to improve vision.

At bedtime, learn to fall asleep with relaxed eyes while listening to music or following your breathing. I recommend massaging and palming the eyes before falling asleep to ensure beginning the next day with relaxed eyes.

BETTE: Cataracts, the clouding of the lens of the eye, is usually treated by surgery. What do you recommend for prevention of cataracts?

JOY: Although the eyes need sunlight for general eye health, cataracts can get worse by too much exposure to UV rays. This accounts for a higher incidence of cataracts in countries closer to the Equator. It is a precautionary measure to wear sunglasses to protect the eyes from UV rays when the sun is excessively bright. That would be the two hours encompassing lunch time in most of North America. Boaters, skiers and drivers need to protect their eyes from the glare of the sun too.

BETTE: Is it at retirement age that most people develop cataracts?

JOY: It is interesting to note that after retirement, people often develop cataracts at a much higher rate then people in their prime working years. I don't accept the idea that cataracts are the natural result of aging. If that were the case, everyone would have cataracts, especially those who spent most of their working life in the sun. Metaphorically speaking, cataracts can signal a clouding of one's view of life, like the inability to see a clear picture of one's future. We could learn something by paying closer attention to who is developing cataracts. Are the cataract patients bored? Unstimulated by their lives? Without definite goals? Emotionally unsatisfied? Unclear as to their direction? Our society has defined the worth of an individual by his/her work role. That is why retirees often cannot perceive a meaningful existence for their future.

BETTE: What can be done to rectify this?

JOY: We could do a lot to change this attitude by realizing that our elders are our biggest natural resource. We should call upon their wisdom, experience and appreciation of life to help us with the collective picture on this planet.

BETTE: What therapies can benefit cataracts?

JOY: The herb bilberry is widely believed to be beneficial in preventing or slowing down the onset of cataracts. Color therapy, especially red and orange filters used on lenses in bright light, helps stimulate the eyes to function more efficiently. Although it is impossible to prove scientifically, I believe this can have a beneficial affect in slowing the development of cataracts, and even preventing them. Also, light practices like sunning, and stimulation of the eyes through exercises, has helped my clients create a whole new, sharper vision for what can be a most rewarding time of life. The incidence of cataracts is much lower in those who know how to care for their eyes. Progress of cataracts is definitely slowed when embracing a natural vision improvement program.

BETTE: Are you in favor of cataract laser surgery even though its long term effects have not been proven?

JOY: It has a fairly good success rate, and post-operative natural vision therapy can maximize the gains. Many elderly people who opt for cataract surgery are not overly concerned about long term effects. They want to see as well as possible in the present time. And a good deal of pleasure is restored by removing the cataract, enabling the person to be more involved in life. Blurred vision can be very frightening and even dangerous to the elderly, so I understand the reasoning in opting for the procedure. Ideally, people should explore natural alternative therapies before resorting to surgery. Each individual must weigh the risks of opting for surgical removal of cataracts. My approach is to teach ways to care for vision to prevent the onset of disease such as cataracts, and to slow its progress if it has begun. I have seen real success with natural vision techniques, but it is difficult to track or measure.

BETTE: What is Macular Degeneration?

JOY: The macula in the eye is the center portion of the retina. It is responsible for central vision, color perception and sharp images. In Macular Degeneration, cone cells of the macula begin to die, reducing the number of cells transmitting visual signals to the brain and decreasing the visual field.

BETTE: Can the disease be slowed up?

JOY: Yes, with light stimulation, color work, rest, visualizations of seeing with clarity and purpose, and reclaiming meaning in life to jump-start energy and promote healing. Also, Leutin, an anti-oxidant, is generally believed to decrease Macular Degeneration. It is found naturally in green leafy vegetables and red peppers, or can be supplemented with 2 or 3 mg. Leutin capsules per day.

BETTE: Are there cures for nervous blinking, shifting and central fixation?

JOY: Blinking is actually good for eye health because it helps keep the muscles fit and relaxed, not still and tense. Also, blinking causes light stimulation. But excessive blinking and twitching are not desirable. Palming has afforded the best results for alleviating these conditions. It is particularly good for central fixation, which is focusing so fully on central space that the periphery is lost. Peripheral awareness can be restored with a procedure I learned from Robert Kaplan. It involves a little device fastened on the bridge of the nose between the eyebrows and covers the inside halves of the eyeballs. This creates a situation where the client sees only the periphery. Utilizing this device for just 15 - 20 minutes twice daily, will help diminish central fixation and relax the whole visual system. A good exercise for correcting eye shifting (eyes that are unable to stay focused) is to bring the thumb towards the nose until the eyes are crossed. This exercise will strengthen muscles and improve concentration and focus. If one eye is very dominant and does most of the focusing work, then this can be done by using a patch so the eyes can be practiced individually as well as together.

BETTE: Would you say that continual headaches may indicate a problem with the eyes?

JOY: Headaches, nausea and dizziness can be caused by many different factors, but can originate from eye problems often rooted in eyestrain.

BETTE: What do you recommend for irritated eyes?

JOY: I suggest keeping an eye pillow in the freezer to place over irritated tired eyes to refresh them at the end of the day. Eye pillows have become popular and can be purchased in gift shops. It is also easy to make one. If you sew a pillow, make it just large enough to be laid over the eyes. The pillow should be made from soft fabric like velvet. Stuff it with flax seed or some light stuffing, and perhaps add lavender or something which has a pleasant scent. Another procedure for alleviating irritated eyes is to lie down, breath deeply, relax and massage the acupressure points on the eyes by gently stimulating the point above and below the corner of the eyes, the center of the eye, the tear ducts and the widest part of the nose. Massaging should always be followed by palming, which is helpful for irritated eyes. Stretching exercises also help. I recommend shoulder shrugging, and bringing the arms around the chest to give yourself a "hug" and open the shoulder blades in the upper back area. Also helpful is bending straight to the side while seated at your desk, allowing your hand to drop to the floor. As you do this, breath deeply to revitalize energy which will soothe irritated eyes.

BETTE: When you do the vision exercises are they done with glasses on or off?

JOY: Always off, or at least, whenever possible. Whenever lenses are not absolutely necessary, it is important to take them off. Minimizing dependency on glasses will stimulate the visual system to work on its own again. We don't need eyeglasses as much as we think we do. Most people can remove them while eating a meal, for example, or having a conversation, listening to music or dancing. The question people should be asking themselves is: "How can I maximize the health of my eyes and become less dependent on my lenses?"

....

Contact Joy Thompson at:

Spirit Centre
106 - West 1st. Street
North Vancouver, BC V7M 1A9
Phone: (604) 904 - 0337
email: joy@spirit-centre.com

RECOMMENDED READING

THE BATES METHOD FOR BETTER EYESIGHT
William Bates
Henry Holt & Co., 1981

TAKE OFF YOUR GLASSES AND SEE
Jacob Liberman
Crown Publishing, 1995

SEEING WITHOUT GLASSES
Robert-Michael Kaplan
Beyond Words Publishing, 1994

THE POWER BEHIND YOUR EYES,
Robert-Michael Kaplan
Inner Traditions International, Ltd., 1995

For tired and irritated eyes, the readings suggest bathing the eyes with a solution of one-third Glyco-Thymoline and two-thirds distilled water.

Eric Mein, MD
From: *KEYS TO HEALTH*

....

8

REFLEXOLOGY
With Melanie B. Shapiro, RN, Reflexologist

....

...and following such a massage, the pressures on the burses in each foot in the achillean burse will relieve the pains in the back and aid the body to sleep. Just indent the finger, forefinger or thumb on the achillean burse from the sole of the foot or heel , you see, and hold it there for two or three minutes-each one, this will release the pressures and relax the body.

EDGAR CAYCE
Reading 632-17

Melanie B. Shapiro, RN, Reflexologist has been a registered nurse for over 14 years, specializing in hospice care. She believes that her near-death experience in October, 2000, heightened her intuitive healing abilities. Shapiro earned certification in Reflexology from the Modern Institute of Reflexology, Lakewood, Colorado. She lives and works in Denver, Colorado.

Reflexology is a holistic healing art. It involves pressure and massage of reflex points such as: the top and bottom of the soles, sides of the feet, palms and the top and sides of the hands. It also includes areas of the ears that stimulate associated organs and functions of the body to increase energy flow and circulation to the pressure points and aroused associated area of the body. For example, when Reflexology techniques are applied to the tips of the toes, which correlates to the head area, the increased flow of energy and circulation causes headaches and sinuses to improve. There are over 40 reflex points in the foot associated with different parts of the anatomy. The same concept applies to the hands and ears, although the ears have more reflex points than the feet and hands.

As a physician and health care educator concerned with preventive medicine methods to naturally enhance the immune system and other self-healing mechanisms, I have become convinced of the value of Reflexology because of my patients' reports of their beneficial responses to this gentle healing art.

William L. Bergman, MD

REFLEXOLOGY
With Melanie B. Shapiro, RN, Reflexologist

Melanie B. Shapiro, RN, Reflexologist, views Reflexology as a type of preventative health maintenance because "... a tender reflex point often indicates a problem arising in the body before the symptoms of the illness ever surface." Sometimes Shapiro finds "congestion", which is a "knot" or hard lump that is not as smooth as muscle should be in the ball of the foot. This condition effects the lung area, and Shapiro views it as indicative of a cold coming on. Her Rx is to apply Reflexology techniques to the congested section on the ball of the foot. This increases energy flow to the lung region, which helps boost the immune system to eliminate the cold. However, Shapiro points out that Reflexology, like many other health care techniques, cannot be effective and/or permanently cure illness if the body continues to be sabotaged by unhealthy lifestyles such as poor diet, lack of exercise, insufficient water intake, and stress related maladies. "I believe that stress is responsible for at least, if not more than 50% of all ailments," Shapiro maintains. "Most people find that Reflexology is very relaxing and helpful for stress."

While Shapiro was a student at Reflexology school, she was taught that Reflexology pressure is often the driving force responsible for flushing out kidney or gallstones from the system. She also learned that the energy being stimulated by Reflexology can induce a pregnant client to go into labor. And she was also taught that pain associated with certain ailments can be eliminated, sometimes forever, with Reflexology.

One of Shapiro's clients was a woman who had chronic pain from rheumatoid arthritis for over 21 years, despite many attempts to find relief through various health techniques and prescriptions. The woman was able to tolerate the Reflexology session, but at the end of her first visit, when she stood up, her foot was so intensely painful that she could hardly walk. "I knew that my client's body was healing and that some temporary physical adjustments were going on to cause this painful reaction," explains Shapiro. A few days later, the woman called to say that she was practically pain free and walking fine for the first time in 21 years. "I'm not sure what this woman's lifestyle was, but I do know that other than her rheumatoid arthritis she was generally healthy," says Shapiro. "Reflexology made the difference in ridding her of pain."

At a Reflexology session, Shapiro massages the foot and hand muscles to dissipate deposits of lactic acid or other minerals known as crystal deposits which cause areas of "congestion". The massage, along with specific pressure techniques on reflex points, stimulates Vital Energy, also known as Chi or the Life Force, circulating between the organs of the body and penetrating every living cell and tissue. Imbalances in the body are rooted in energy blockages that occur when crystal deposits formulate in portions of the hands or feet, (there is not enough muscle tissue in the ears for crystal deposits to roost) which are connected to the tissue balanced areas of the body. When the residue is broken down, energy blockages dissipate and endorphins are probably released, because the joy and relaxation that takes place indicates this to be so.

"To prove that endorphins are released is difficult, because Reflexology is energy based and can't be measured outside laboratory/research settings," Shapiro points out. "But stimulated nerve endings and pressure points in the feet, hands and ears have been observed countless times to influence self-healing in related unbalanced areas of the body." She says that people easily feel the breakdown of abrasive crystal deposits as they become smoother, and the circulation and lymphatic system flows fluidly. The result is that toxins are released into the bloodstream. A lot of water is required to flush the poisons from the system. Shapiro recommends drinking at least 12 glasses of water a day, which is 4 more glasses then usually prescribed.

She likes doing at least five minutes of Reflexology per session on the ears because it is so soothing to the client and can affect a greater area of the body, since the ears contain more reflex points than the hands and feet. "At each session, I usually stimulate a client's brain activity in the brain/pituitary area by activating the reflex point at the top/center of the ear lobe."

When Shapiro locates an area of discomfort at a reflex point, it signals her to work that zone so the body can heal in the associated ailing portion of the anatomy. "Usually, the pain lessens. But if there is unusual unrelenting pain, I refer the client to a physician for diagnosis and treatment," she says.

The Egyptian culture recorded the use of Reflexology as early as 2330 BC. Other ancient texts reveal that Chinese, Japanese, Indian and Russian people also worked on the feet to encourage good health. Reflexology as we know it today was first introduced to the USA in 1913 by Dr. William Fitzgerald. "At that time Reflexology was a painful experience, but that is not the case today," says Shapiro. Modern Reflexology relies on natural forces of the body to heal itself once it is impelled by reflex stimulation. Shapiro was trained to use lasers, air hammers and many other hand tools, but prefers the healing energy in her hands for Reflexology. The only time she uses hand tools is when she is unable to reach a pressure point deeply enough with her fingers.

One of the home healing energy techniques that Shapiro recommends is applying lotion to the top and bottom of the hands and feet. Pressing anywhere on the top and bottom of the hands and feet will exert pressure that stimulates energy to those points and their associated body areas. "You don't have to be a Reflexologist to do this," she says. Sometimes Shapiro does Reflexology on hospice patients, with the intent of providing supportive palliative treatment. "It is very comforting for them because it feels so good."

....

As Reflexologists, we want to be known as givers and sustainers of life.
We are called to guide the seeker into wellness of body, mind, soul and spirit.

Zachary Brinkerhoff, Reflexologist
President and Director of Studies
at the Modern Institute of Reflexology

....

Contact Melanie B. Shapiro, RN, Reflexologist at:
menemab333@home.com

....

RECOMMENDED BOOKS

FEET FIRST:
A Guide To Foot Reflexology
Laura Norman
Fireside , 1988

ACUPRESSURE:
Ancient Wisdom for Modern-Day Healing
Monte Cunningham
New Age Press, 1994

BODY REFLEXOLOGY:
Healing at Your Fingertips
Mildred Carter et al
Prentice Hall Press, 2002

ILLUSTRATED GUIDE TO
FULL BODY REFLEXOLOGY
Barbara Dodd
Woodland Publishing Incorporated, 1996

HOW TO FIND A REFLEXOLOGIST IN YOUR AREA

1. Consult the Yellow Pages under "Reflexology".

***

2. Use your Internet search engines to obtain information on Reflexologists or Reflexology Associations in your area.

***

3. Contact the Reflexology Association of America:
402 S. Rainbow Blvd., Las Vegas, NV 89103-2059

Phone: 702-871-9522

***

4. Contact the International Council of Reflexologists, Canada:
PO Box 30513, Richmond Hill, Ontario L4COC7, Canada
Phone: 1-800-221-7963
Fax: 1-905-884-0294

....

9

THE HEALING POWER OF GEMSTONES
Interview With William Stuber, Gem Therapist

....

We would then find that the one (stone) that is the nearer in accord to the vibrations of the body that may use same would be the more effective with that particular body. Yet the very nature of the thing (stone) makes it effective with -any - body, you see; but the more effective with one that is in accord, or whose positive and negative vibrations are according with the stone itself, see? for it (the stone) throws off as well as draws in...through the positive-negative vibration...

EDGAR CAYCE
Reading 440-18

William Stuber, author, teacher and coach for practitioners of gemstone healing, is one of the foremost healers currently employing gems as a tool to encourage better health physically, mentally, emotionally and spiritually. He utilizes a selection of eight gems and his own unique diamond therapy techniques. Stuber facilitates workshops and classes on gem healing for beginners and practitioners. He authored *Gems of the 7 Color Rays* (Llewellyn Publications, 2001). His book covers many aspects of gem healing, employing a color ray model for differentiating gems into categories and drawing broad generalizations about their properties and uses.

....

...it is necessary that there be...the analysis of the composition of the stones as related to their vibrations-as relate then to a human body, see? ...the vibrations being those that are of the positive and negative natures in the very stone itself...

EDGAR CAYCE
Reading 440-18

....

INTERVIEW WITH WILLIAM STUBER, GEM THERAPIST

BETTE: For what purposes, besides decoration, are gemstones used?

WILLIAM: Gemstones are amazing compact vibrational color energy tools. With proper intent, they can help attune a person to their natural healing abilities through the Creative Forces to restore balance to the physical, mental, emotional and spiritual systems.

BETTE: Can healing take place if there is great damage to the tissues?

WILLIAM: If it is not too great, the body easily heals itself with the correct vibrational information. Gemstone healing can help the body expel harmful toxins which it holds by attraction (negative vibrations attract other negative vibrations). Add proper dietary and exercise practices and it is possible to regain excellent health.

BETTE: Do all metals, stones and gems have the same vibrational ability to aid in healing?

WILLIAM: They have various inherent vibrational characteristics. Gems like citrine, zincite, tourmaline, quartz and topaz provide highly concentrated oscillation that can change existing detrimental vibrations in the body. They grow naturally and are crystalline in structure. Some have consistent color and form, according to the precise alignment of their molecules. Other gemstones are grown by sea creatures, or formed like fossils in the process of mineralization or under heat pressure. Most gemstones were originally shaped or formed crystals and are used as adornments or healing tools. But stones that are a conglomerate form, like jasper or any sedimentary or metamorphic rock, are considerably less formidable in their potential for healing. Metals like gold, silver or lead and other pure inorganic form substances mined out of the ground, purified by fire or separated from the ore they were formed in, are even less active than stones. This is especially so if they have been melted down and formed into shapes. Metals do not contact the inner healer the way gems do.

BETTE: But the composition of gems, stones and minerals in regard to their vibrations have some likelihood of use as healing tools for the human body?

WILLIAM: Yes, when used in solutions with water, oil and derivatives from plants. The key to unlocking the mystery of their use is knowing how to prescribe them, when to use what, in which way to use it and for how long. All answers, however, are within the inner healer and exhibit themselves through the body's positive or negative vibrational reactions.

BETTE: I understand that the same vibrational healing imparted by gemstones can be accomplished with homeopathic medicines, herbs, charged water, sound/music and other vibrations.

WILLIAM: That is true, but I believe that Gem Therapy is the most penetrating, highly effective, subtle form of vibrational healing.

BETTE: Do people react similarly to the healing power of gemstones?

WILLIAM: Reactions to high levels of gemstone color energy vary from person to person. This is dependent upon how the flow of energy moves or does not move in the body, mind, emotions and spirit. Vibrational patterns of stones are known to change according to the interaction between the client and gemstone therapist. However, gemstone vibrations are adjustable by the practitioner within a certain range. To accomplish this, intensive training and focused intention are necessary to direct energy and vibrational patterns of the gems into areas of the body requiring adjustment. A gentle assurance and tone, along with the correct vibration, will cause a shift in the ailing area. Of course, ultimately, it is the intuition of the inner healer that knows which gemstone vibration is needed to encourage profound healing in the body.

BETTE: A number of Edgar Cayce's readings recommended certain colors of stones for raising vibrations in the body. In reading 3806 - 1, for example, he talks about utilizing the purple to bluish violet color of the amethyst for restraining the disposition: ***"In the choice of stones, do wear the amethyst as a pendant about the neck, as part of the jewelry. This will also work with the colors to control temperament."*** How do other colors of gemstones influence the human condition?

WILLIAM: Color vibrations are very powerful: I use: violet gemstones to affect the subconscious and the higher consciousness, indigo to fortify the intuition, blue to enhance the mind/consciousness and sense apparatus, green to empower the heart and physical health, orange to cause impromptu memories of karma, red to influence emotions, yellow to strengthen the spirit, and white to integrate all of these elements and enhance the soul.

BETTE: In your book *Gems Of The 7 Color Rays* you include a detailed selection of 58 stones suitable for healing. Did you write about every common gemstone available?

WILLIAM: I chose those that are most likely to be available in excellent quality and have the capability of healing most common afflictions produced by conflicts in the energy field. Stones that I have not listed can be found in *Crystal Communion* or any books by Melody.

BETTE: Are gems meant to be worn in certain ways to benefit from their healing energies?

WILLIAM: They can be worn as necklaces when one wishes to infuse the whole body with gem energy. But wearing a single stone on a specific point on the body can be even more powerful for healing a small area. To change the body's energy, it is important to use only excellent quality stones.

BETTE: Is it necessary to wear a gemstone to reap its healing benefits, or will close proximity to the gemstone be equally helpful?

WILLIAM: Placing a single gem near the bedside will afford excellent results in accessing dreams and developing a spiritual connection with Ascendant Masters and angels, beings who offer advice, love and support to the seeker of healing.

BETTE: What is the purpose of altering the natural crystalline shape of gemstones into rounded and spherical shapes?

WILLIAM: The energy surrounding a natural crystalline shape of a gem is quite forceful. It can cause stress and injury to an individual in its presence. By softening the gem to a rounded or spherical shape, a gentle but constant infusion of energy is transmitted to those in its proximity. A sphere's energetic power can gradually and gently nourish the body, encouraging it to heal and rebuild its strength. The energy flowing around a spherical gem only enters the body when it draws on it, as opposed to the stress of forceful entry characteristic of the overpowering gem energy emitted from naturally occurring shapes.

BETTE: Several of Cayce's readings suggested that by wearing something made of carbon steel metal, on oneself or in a groin pocket, the body would be ionized, ***"...from it's very vibrations - to resist cold, congestion and those inclinations for disturbance with the mucous membranes of the throat and nasal passages."*** (1842-1). Which gemstones, crystals or metals do you implement to alleviate specific aliments?

WILLIAM: I have placed large spheres on the body to clear disharmony and reduce the effects of chaos and conflict exhibited in a client's aura. This helps with emotional and mental aberrations by reducing stress and alleviating or minimizing the effects of trauma. Small crystals are effective for minute body adjustments. They can be used in chiropractic care by manipulating the lines of force used in traditional Eastern medicine, which can be traced and adjusted with training but are not visible to the untrained eye. The lines of force directly control body posture as well as cellular changes affecting an increase in water flow in the body, adjustment of electromagnetic forces, reduction of toxicity, improvement of cellular reproduction and returning a function to its original purpose.

BETTE: Are crystals and gemstones useful in changing the energy of a space?

WILLIAM: Crystals and natural formed shapes of coral, amber, jasper and agate work best for implementing energy change of a space where Fung Shui design is applied.

BETTE: What do you recommend for changing the whole body vibration?

WILLIAM: The use of gemstones like aventurine in a full tub of bath water so there is maximum body contact with gemstone energy. By doing this, in most cases, the body will immediately recognize foreign substances hidden within the cells, eliminate them and turn off body alarms. The result will be eradication of stress, pain and discomfort. Citrine is also excellent for this purpose.

BETTE: Will Gem Therapy help remove the effects of past life trauma or trauma to the body in general?

WILLIAM: A trained gem therapist can reduce, but not completely get rid of, past life traumas. Gemstone healing is highly effective in restoring energetic flow patterns due to a simple fall or blow to the body. It is important to know that even a mild accident can create ongoing damage disruptive to the sensitive flow of life energy. A mild accident can cause future health problems.

BETTE: How effective is remote Gem Therapy?

WILLIAM: Gems definitely revise conditions for the person at a distance. I place gemstones upon a surrogate, choosing gems required to psychically understand what is happening physically, mentally, emotionally and spiritually in the remote person. In turn, this affects the receiver and allows me to view their reactions. As a result of the active reading, I am able to suggest to the remote person which stones are applicable to their body for self-healing. This form of reading is highly effective.

BETTE: Would you give an example of the dynamics that take place in a client that you have helped remotely?

WILLIAM: Once I was called by a woman suffering from a variety of emotional disorders, including occasional paranoia, paranormal hearing of voices and inability to hold a job. During her two remote sessions, I recorded intuitive information that I received from her guides. It concerned abuse she suffered by her father and emotional abandonment by her mother. I also recorded specific suggestions given by my guides and observations of her childhood. And I observed an increase in overall energy from the placement of gemstones on the surrogate. I intuitively sensed her thoughts, emotions and inner knowledge of what to do about her state of health. To help her discover her true feelings and memories of the past without fearing them, I guided my focused intent into a crystal ball. This process amplified and directed my verbal suggestions, telepathic visualizations, direct aura adjustment and resonance (an action that produces an observable affect). It was also responsible for guidance of her electromagnetic flux in a different direction and reduced wave-like vibrations of her individual points where maladjustment of her inner energy field reached a point of crisis in her body. I channeled information from her inner soul awareness to clear a path for her eventual healing.

BETTE: Did the process result in her instant health improvement?

WILLIAM: There was an immediate release of pent up emotions, clearing of chaotic thought patterns, reduction of pain, movement where there was none and improved posture. Her conflict resolution within her emotional body initiated her recovery. Within several months she was able to make peace with herself, and her old resentment and pain disappeared along with her major symptoms.

BETTE: Do you possess special divine healing powers?

WILLIAM: I am only a facilitator who aids individuals in accessing and communicating with the intrinsic healer inside themselves. My purpose is to use Gem Therapy to facilitate an awareness of personal potential to self-heal. I use stones as a tool to release emotions, open areas of tension, ease pain, heighten energy flow, reduce inflammation and detoxify the body.

BETTE: Edgar Cayce stated in reading 707-2 that the higher purpose of using gem shapes and natural materials is to attune with the Christ Consciousness. Is this your ultimate purpose as a gemstone healer?

WILLIAM: Cayce's reading embraces my higher purpose. I also believe that every person has a life direction of their own choosing. Gems have helped me find my higher purpose in life and have brought me into companionship with Source. My inner guides have helped me discover my life as a healer, skilled observer and one who can intuitively sense energy disturbances and read auras. I can also "feel" another person's body sensations, and "see" details of their past lives with "inner eyes", as one would see a memory.

BETTE: What past incarnations have you had that affect your present life's work?

WILLIAM: I was one of the individuals who helped set up the original configurations in Atlantis. This allowed for transportation of solid objects to help control certain mental disorders. The crystals that were used by certain government agencies were disrupting peace and tranquillity in the world. To offset the symptomatic disruptions in the consciousness of the people of Atlantis, we built large stone structures to help balance the energy to a certain degree. The government's use of crystals disrupted the earth's energy field. Unknown to me at the time, people in power seized the technology for manipulation of mankind. Their misuse of this advanced system of knowledge was responsible for major earth movements that eventually submerged the continent of Atlantis. These individuals are presently reincarnated and continue to be power-hungry, greedy and self-exalting, putting the world at dangerous risk of annihilation.

BETTE: What can be done to prevent this?

WILLIAM: Nothing, unless violence is exerted, a measure I do not endorse. Each of us, however, will reap what we sow. Every person has a choice in raising the earth's vibrational level by healing self.

BETTE: When discussing the approach to psychic experience by way of gem vibrations, Cayce cautioned that if gemstones were used for selfish purposes they would ***"turn and rend..." the user.*** What are the dangers of using gemstones?

WILLIAM: Without operating in accordance with the laws of love, the high vibrational energy of gemstones creates a new harm that ricochets back to the energy sender with a vengeance. You will be safe when using gemstones by giving love freely, without the intent of seeking control or limiting the way others use this love.

BETTE: What other options are there besides using your intuition for choosing the right stones, gems and metals for healing?

WILLIAM: Muscle testing, which is known as kinesiology, is another option. It involves holding a muscle in its fully extended position and testing for its average strength. The procedure involves gripping a stone in the hand not being muscle tested, or holding a clear thought of that particular stone, or placing the stone on your lap and at the same time testing the strength of the fully extended arm muscle. A strong arm that holds its strength when challenged will indicate a positive response to the stone. If the extended arm is weak, it indicates that the stone is not correct for helping the healing.

BETTE: Is there any way to get a more precise answer to a question like: "Can this stone help relieve stress in my jaw?"

WILLIAM: Hold the stone up to your jaw and ask yourself the question. At the same time, see if the fully extended arm not holding the stone remains strong or is weakened in response to downward pressure. You will be unable to hold your arm out if your body is answering "no" to the posed question. "No" indicates that the jaw needs a different stone to jump-start self-healing.

BETTE: Do you teach your students kinesiology among other things?

WILLIAM: I teach a subtle method of kinesiology to students which requires a quiet mind and clear focus. And I also teach the art of placing the correctly chosen healing stone, the expected outcome, which size, shape, color and clarity to use, the ideal time of placement and the length of treatment. Stones can be placed using a metallic holder, string, chain or tape. Also, stones can be placed in a nylon or cloth bag that is affixed to the body. Some of this information is available through Ayurvedic or western astrology methods.

BETTE: Why did some of Cayce's readings suggest that certain stones be worn around the waist or other parts of the body?

WILLIAM: Wearing a gemstone over the area of the body where the problem exists would be the best place to start healing with a gem. A string with an attached gem worn around the waist might be just the thing to relieve tension in that area. The waist is where numerous problems are stored by many individuals.

BETTE: Are birthstones strictly symbolic, or are they carriers of particular energy associated with certain months?

WILLIAM: All birthstones are powerful carriers of color healing energy and can be used for good purpose. Certain gems, like emerald, sapphire and diamond possess more power than other birthstones. Pearl, for example, is less powerful, and is not really a stone or a gem. Ultimately, the means to getting excellent results with any gemstone lies in the intent of its use.

BETTE: But does one's birthstone have more healing power to cure one's ailments than other gemstones?

WILLIAM: If you wish to understand yourself better, then, by all means, use the stone associated with your birth month. For answers to deeper questions concerning the purpose of your existence, explore the symbolism of your birthstone, which lies in its shape, color, location where it was found and other physical properties of the stone. Information can be accessed by allowing these vibrational "stone people", as native Americans refer to them, to tell you what you need to know through your dreams or higher consciousness.

BETTE: Where does one begin with gemstone healing?

WILLIAM: Once the question of what to heal is ascertained by muscle testing, or choosing what you wish to address, the process of experimenting and verifying begins with the use of gemstones. Using one's intuition coupled with skills from whatever approach you are familiar with, whether it is Acupuncture,

Chiropractic or Gem Therapy, will accomplish safe healing and guide you to deeper levels of interaction with gemstones.

BETTE: Which gemstones should a beginner experiment with first?

WILLIAM: Start with only a few stones, like black onyx or leopardskin jasper, to protect or ground yourself. Good choices for the inexperienced user are: clear quartz or citrine for improving health, amethyst to heal the affects of false self-image, and rhodonite, rhodocrosite or ruby for emotional healing. Learning about your reaction to the energy of various stones can be a cornerstone in the process of eliminating emotional baggage, which is essential for realizing good health. In general, it is best to find a qualified Gem Therapist to teach you how to become attuned to the healing power of gems and their deeper purpose for discerning self-realization.

BETTE: Where can stones, gems and metals be obtained?

WILLIAM: Sometimes you can get them from your Gem Therapy teacher. And there are three suppliers of therapeutic gemstones that I recommend: Gemisphere in Portland, Oregon, Lightstreams in Seattle, Washington, and Visioneering in Carlsborg, Washington, which is my company. *(See end of chapter for contact information.)*

BETTE: Why not go to a regular jewelry store for stones, gems and metals?

WILLIAM: I don't recommend jewelry stores for the novice. He/she should look for good quality in gemstones without paying a fortune. Part of the power of gemstones is the excellence of the material and the precision of the manufacture of bead, sphere, or shaped crystal, as well as its vibrational characteristics. If you are not sure about what these terms mean or how to assess the therapeutic quality of a gem, go to a qualified reputable gem specialty store, like the ones I mentioned. They will show you a fine assortment of gems so you get optimum results when you implement gem healing. You can, however, safely buy metals from any honest jeweler. Although the price may be high for platinum or gold, the quality can be trusted because it is government standardized.

BETTE: So quality is more important than quantity?

WILLIAM: Owning large quantities of expensive gems will not provide nearly as much benefit as owning one quality gemstone and knowing how to use it to access information from your higher self. A small gem of excellent quality will out-perform a large gem of poor or mixed quality where the material is uneven and parts of it contain inclusions.

BETTE: Can a gem therapist teach you to access your inner healer?

WILLIAM: Yes, a qualified gem therapist, or a school for Gem Therapy like Lightstreams in Seattle or Gemisphere in Portland, can show you how to access your inner healer with the use of high quality gemstones. Also, a psychic can retrieve this information for you from his/her inner guide or from your own inner guide. The techniques for self-healing that I teach to practitioners enable them to utilize gems with other healing practices to encourage self-healing.

BETTE: What if a qualified gemstone teacher is not available?

WILLIAM: Then use your intuition to guide you in the choice of gemstones for healing, but do it with a realistic sense of your capabilities. As a beginner, you cannot expect to attain miraculous results with Gem Therapy. Also, remember to practice your intent, without using force, to communicate with the Divine.

BETTE: Do you utilize the knowledge of gemstones that ancient cultures tapped into?

WILLIAM: Not really. Very old cultures used stones in magical ways, quite differently than the way stones are used today. Unlike our ancestors, we often miss the magic of the way spirit moves. Ancient people, and the vibrational strength of their stones, were of a different consciousness than ours because their life energy was slower in pace and more agrarian. Also, their populations were smaller and more primitive.

Many ancient cultures like the Mayans, Egyptians and Atlanteans used their knowledge of stones and metals for destruction of, or influence over, their enemies, with amplification of psychic powers. Rarely do I try to move energy by force. I primarily use gemstone knowledge I have garnered through experimentation, research and observation of the dynamic affects of stones. Most of my work is based on what the stones intuitively tell me to do in terms of placement on a particular point of the body. I also am sensitive to their message of resonating differently than usual in proximity to a diseased area of the body, or when they gain vibrational power in proximity to a healthy organ. I rely on my observations of actual changes in the stones and the resulting movement, jerking, heating, cooling and emotional release from the treated body.

BETTE: What stones did the ancients use?

WILLIAM: Malachite, opal, moonstone, ruby, emerald, sardonyz/carnelian, agate, garnet, lapis lazuli, lapis linguis and certain metals including copper. Some were ground into powder, others were shaped and many were cut and mounted. Stones like lapis lazuli and metals like copper have lost their potency, to a considerable extent, and are not available in their crystal or gem form at this time.

BETTE: Have any new stones been discovered?

WILLIAM: Hundreds of new stones are available today that were unheard of in ancient times. I use a number of new stones in my own newly devised therapies including: sugulite from Africa, phrenite from Madagascar, charorite from Russia, and danburite from North America. I have found that new stones carry new wisdom to utilize in contemporary society.

BETTE: How are the new stones more effective than the old ones?

WILLIAM: New stones have been created by the earth to help the planet deal with immense pressures generated by modern technology, prolonged use of high electromagnetic fields and ecologically harmful chemicals. New stones are also able to adjust more varieties of harmful aberrations, such as those formed in cancerous tissues that have been exposed to toxins and grow excessively out of control.

BETTE: Are you currently involved in doing any research with gemstones?

WILLIAM: I work with a group of alternative health care practitioners who utilize Gem Therapy in conjunction with Massage, Chiropractic, Cranial Sacral, Touch for Health, Therapeutic Touch, Reiki, Shin Jitsu, Chi Gung, Tai Chi, Acupressure, Acupuncture, Polarity Therapy and other healing techniques that remove stagnation and restore a healthy flow of energy to the body. We have found that Gem Therapy, combined with other modalities that move energy through the physical body, helps people adapt more gracefully to the physical, mental, emotional and spiritual changes that take place when vibrational energy is restoring the body to a stasis. Our group has also been researching dimensions that overlap ours, like the astral plane which is similar to the earth plane. But the astral plane is of a higher vibration so it is not visible to the physical eye, although it can be experienced through spiritual work. Modern physics suggests that the existence of other dimensions is proven mathematically. The group I am working with wishes to contact Ascendant Masters of Gem Therapy, on the astral plane, for their secrets of healing. By obtaining this information, we can all experience better health and enjoy our planet for higher purposes than war, greed, poverty, pestilence, perversion, obsession, power and other dark passions of the mind.

BETTE: The great spiritual teacher Paramhansa Yogananda said: *"Pearls and other jewels, as well as metals and plants, applied directly to the human skin, exercise an electromagnetic influence over the physical cells. Man's body contains carbon and various metallic elements that are present also in plants, metals and jewels. The discovery of the rishis in these fields will doubtless receive confirmation some day from physiologists..."* Have scientists confirmed Yogananda's words?

WILLIAM: Few scientists are devoted to the work pioneered by mystics suggesting that energy is the key to good health. Fortunately, we can rely on, and learn from those special individuals who look deeply into the mysteries of energy and see the truth. The affects of gemstones are many, including: electrical, electromagnetic, resonance, color, light, harmonic and vibrational (as in homeopathy), spin/directional (reversing the spin on atoms) and kinetic which applies to all energy of motion.

BETTE: Cayce suggested an experiment for a person seeking a reading in which he said: ***"Go to the New York Museum of Natural History. Sit by a large quantity of this type of stone (lapis) and listen and sing! Do it in the open! Don't let others make a fool of you, or their remarks overcome you, but sit by it and listen at it sing: for it does! It's from Arizona."*** (440-3 (9). Have you ever heard a stone sing?

WILLIAM: All stones have a certain vibrational sound. Some individuals, like me, can easily hear it as a kind of music or melody of life. In certain large deposits of material of exceptional quality, the sound is particularly lovely and will uplift the soul. Arizona has many such large deposits, but so do other locations around the planet. I highly recommend visiting some of these spots like Herkimer mines, Brazilian mines, or mines in Arkansas, California and Montana to enjoy the music. Incidentally, some people experience this vibrational music as thought, light, a feeling in the body, emotions and rhythmical patterns. Also, singing is an excellent therapy, especially to the accompaniment of natural sounds of gems, waterfalls and other natural phenomena, to relax tension and focus the mind on more pleasant thoughts that bring one in touch with the spiritual aspect of life.

BETTE: In your book *Gems of the 7 Color Rays,* it says that you have mastered the use of gemstones to clear weakness. What weakness are you referring to?

WILLIAM: Weakness is the feeling you have when your energy is low for any reason, and your mental sharpness, vitality, power, raw emotional drive and physical stamina are not up to par. Ongoing untreated weakness will result in stagnation of physical, mental, emotional and spiritual energy, and atrophy will quickly set in. To bring up energy on all levels of the system, it is necessary to exercise the energy centers of the body with therapeutic gemstones. Gems can provide nutritional color ray energy to detoxify the body and return it to normal balance. Also, weakness should be treated by increasing nutritional supply with green vegetables rich in minerals in their organic form.

BETTE: What is Diamond Therapy?

WILLIAM: It's a sophisticated application of gemstones that is possible only with the highest quality diamonds proven to contain the precise color ray spectrum required for work with the human genetic code. Diamond Therapy is the most profound and fundamental way of altering the response patterns we operate within. It can gradually and comfortably aid in gaining complete control over the entire function of the system to allow the inner healer to heal the body.

BETTE: Can a gemstone novice learn Diamond Therapy?

WILLIAM: I do not recommend it for beginners. Only a few therapeutic diamonds have been discovered. To the best of my knowledge, there is no one who is working at this time to successfully grade diamonds. I was fortunate enough to have been psychically directed by discarnate entities, who are guardians of diamond energy, to obtain several of these special diamonds. Specific instructions were given on how to use them to dramatically alter the energy flow patterns across the astral bodies. This includes our physical, mental and emotional states. Normally, the physical, mental and emotional bodies occupy the same relative space and are hard to differentiate. However, each of these bodies can exist separately. For example, the mental body can live on even though the physical body dies.

BETTE: How do you integrate Diamond Therapy with other gemstone techniques to help the body regain health?

WILLIAM: To begin with, I use color ray therapies employing gemstone strands of spherical beads to settle the turbulence in the aura caused by emotional conflict. Using small spheres taped to particular points on the body, I discharge energy that is not purely physical. Next, I realign the astral bodies by adjusting the flow of subtle energies between the physical, mental and emotional bodies with the use of medium sized spheres. This is followed by small crystals of many different colors which energize points where the flow has been constricted. Then I utilize Diamond Therapy to adjust the chakras by attuning the petals, separate pathways of energy flowing within these centers, to a central harmonic resonance between two or more resonant vibrations that the treated person intuitively feels is healthy.

BETTE: It seems like an intricate procedure.

WILLIAM: It is; and there's more. When I complete the process I just described, I remove blockages by repairing rents in the auric field through the steady application of infused energy, until the body repairs itself. Then I invite visiting entities to leave the body. When the electromagnetic field is restored, communications between the various parts of the body reconnect. Finally, I adjust the control centers in the brain by reprogramming thousands of energy flow points to produce the best possible health throughout the system, given the condition of its physical structure. After all these steps are completed, I use Diamond Therapy again to clear any remaining problematic non-color ray energies. Conditions would then be correct for the person I am treating to receive even deeper levels of Diamond Therapy that reprogram energy centers so they can follow their natural functions.

BETTE: Are there cases where Diamond Therapy cannot correct negative conditions?

WILLIAM: I have found there are very few cases where conditions are irreversible and cannot move into spontaneous remission.

BETTE: You are saying that major improvements, in health, attitude, self-image, psychic abilities, spiritual integrity, joy and other positive emotional responses, are likely with these reprogramming techniques?

WILLIAM: The new use of energy, along with exercise and a healthy diet, will give almost everyone's inner healer the necessary tools to transform the physical, mental and emotional bodies to a healthier condition. At times there is a need for allopathic medicine. And many conditions require multiple methods of healing for correction. But, in general, the new use of energy is equivalent to operations in a computer. Each function can be corrected and new ones developed with the right software, so the hardware can operate according to its original intent. Change your energy patterns, and you can change your life.

....

RECOMMENDED READING

GEMS OF THE 7 COLOR RAYS
William Stuber
Lewellyn Publications, 2001

GEMS AND STONES
Based on the Edgar Cayce Readings
A.R.E. Press, 1979

CRYSTALLINE COMMUNION
Colleen Marquist and Jack Frasl
Earthlight, 1999

GIFTS OF THE GEMSTONE GUARDIANS
Michael and Jimmy Katz
Gemisphere, 1989

Schools for The Study of Gem Therapy and Suppliers of Therapeutic Gemstones

Visioneering
PO Box 21
Carlsborg, WA 98324
Phone: 1-866-681-8485

Lightstreams
3272 California Ave. SW
Seattle WA 98116
Phone: 1-877-321-4383

Gemisphere
2812 N. W. Thurman
Portland OR 97210
Phone: 503-241-3642

....

The gate of stone is the gateway to spiritual and psychic advancement through the correct use of stones and gems. Stones and gems are tools that aid in our search for betterment of our lives on all levels.

DJ Conway
From: *CRYSTAL ENCHANTMENTS*

....

For a reading, personal training session
or gemstone tutoring program
contact William Stuber at:

William Stuber c/o
Visioneering
PO Box 21
Carlsborg, WA 98324
360-681-8485

or toll free when ordering supplies:
866-681-8485
williamstube@surfbest.net

As to stones, have near to self, wear preferably upon the body about the neck, the lapis lazuli; this preferably encased in crystal. It will be not merely as an ornament, but as strength from the emanation which will be gained by the body always from same. For the stone is itself an emanation of vibrations of the elements that give vitality, virility, strength, and that of assurance in self.

EDGAR CAYCE
Reading 1981-1

10

SHOPPING FOR HEALTH AT THE A.R.E. HOUSTON CENTER COMPLEX
A Tour With Ed Jamail and Carl Bohannon

....

Castor oil taken internally and such eliminants are only purgatives. Hence the castor oil absorbed from the packs will be better than taking same internally.

EDGAR CAYCE
Reading 1433-6

(The Violet Ray)..would be to create a balance of circulation through the superficial portion of the body, causing a bettering of the conditions.

EDGAR CAYCE
Reading 436-4

Ed Jamail is the former owner of Jamail's Market, a well-known landmark in Houston. Jamail has been involved in Edgar Cayce's work since 1968. During that year he had major surgery which resulted in his near-death experience. Following his surgical recovery, Jamail met some A.R.E. members who explained his near-death experience to him from a Cayce perspective. They recommended that he read about Cayce; after doing so, Jamail began to incorporate Cayce's philosophy into his own life. He became so well-versed with Cayce's readings that he has been able to use his acquired knowledge to guide many people in finding Cayce-related answers to alleviate their health problems. Jamail is Chairman of the Board for the Houston Search for God Council, and Coordinator of the new A.R.E. Houston Center Complex. He served the A.R.E. on a national level as a member of the Board of Trustees. Jamail has also administered at the local level for the Houston Search For God Council, and in the Southwest Region as well. He has lectured about Edgar Cayce throughout North America, Africa, Germany and the Near East, where he started many A.R.E. Search For God Study Groups.

Carl Leon Bohannon, co-director of the A.R.E. Houston Center Complex, was introduced to metaphysics and Edgar Cayce by his father in the early 1960s. Ever since then, Bohannon has been a student of dreams, meditation and healing. His career in commercial design and an interest in science and spirituality has culminated in his current involvement with the Houston A.R.E. Center Complex. Bohannon writes and lectures nationwide on spirituality and healing, specializing in the use of color, sound and meditation for rejuvenating the physical body. Teaching others how to heal their lives with all of God's healing tools is his passion.

The activity on this is not only for the destruction of live tubercule tissue, but it (Charred Oak Keg 100% Apple Brandy) acts as an antiseptic for all irritated areas; also giving activity to cellular force of the corpuscle itself. It acts as a stimuli to the circulation, then, recharging each cell as it passes through areas so affected by the radiation of the gases from this fluid itself.

EDGAR CAYCE
Reading 3176-1

SHOPPING FOR HEALTH AT THE A.R.E. HOUSTON CENTER COMPLEX

A Tour With Ed Jamail and Carl Bohannon

Several months ago, I visited the A.R.E. Houston Search For God Council's new Center Complex. It is located on 1.5 acres of land in a 17,000 square foot warehouse, at 7800 Amelia, Houston, Texas. Many years of hard work by Houston area study group members, coordinated by the Search For God Council, Inc., a non-profit corporation, have resulted in bringing the legacy of Edgar Cayce's vision to Houston. The spiritual ideal and goal for the Center is to reach out to spiritual seekers with encouragement and support, and to facilitate God's will and work. Ed Jamail and Carl Bohannon, longtime members and lecturers for the A.R.E, manage the Center. It is open to the public to investigate metaphysics and experiment with many healing remedies suggested by Edgar Cayce.

"After much prayer and meditation, we realized that buying the property was the right thing to do," said Jamail. In '96 and '97 A.R.E. Houston drew a total of 1500 people to their Holistic Exposition held at the University of Houston. "That's when we decided a Center was needed so people could come on a regular basis to learn about the work of Edgar Cayce and have access to the numerous remedies he spoke of in his readings," Jamail explained.

They began with a workshop presented by Carl Bohannon to create an ideal for a Center. The operative principle was to set the spiritual ideal for a Center and then let "spirit arrange the rest," explained Jamail. At the workshop, participants formulated messages for a subliminal tape. Thirty volunteers agreed to record the tape in their own voices and play it back for three weeks as they went about their daily routines. Some of the messages delivered to their consciousness were: "We love our new A.R.E. Center."; "It will be easy to obtain the Center."; "The Center's energy is very good." Within eight months, Houston A.R.E. opened a one room Center in an extra office donated by Dixie, USA, which is owned by two A.R.E. members. The Center sold books about Edgar Cayce and remedies and apparatuses mentioned in his readings.

After 18 months, Dixie, USA had outgrown the facility and needed larger headquarters. When they offered to sell A.R.E. the building and acreage, Jamail and A.R.E. Houston called upon Mary Roach, a gifted intuitive and long-time A.R.E. member, to do a reading about the Center. Her Source said that the project was a gift from God. Roach advised the A.R.E. to buy the premises. She informed them that an amazing amount of help and money was forthcoming. They decided to purchase the property and began organizing a fund-raiser to generate cash for purchase of the premises.

Many people volunteered their help, including two graphic designers who were members of a study group. Their company, Vilven Designs, created an unusual mailer in the form of a three-dimensional pyramid shaped paper sculpture. Each section of the pyramid contained descriptive copy and illustrations of the Center's project. The response to this mailer was phenomenal. People began sending donations and in six months $150,000 was raised. A.R.E Headquarters in Virginia Beach loaned an additional $50,000 for the down payment to purchase the property and start remodeling.

Roach did a "check-up" reading on the Center six months before it opened. She commented on how ambitious the plans had become and advised that 90% of the goals would be achieved. Her reading also determined that the Center would attract major media attention, making its objectives achievable. Subsequently, several companies and individuals inquired about doing video taping at the Center and a production studio has even begun discussions about relocating their facilities to the premises.

Jamail and Bohannon invited me to tour the spacious Center. There was an area with an expanded bookstore stocking all Cayce related material in English and Spanish. Well-known authors were represented on the shelves on topics relating to metaphysics. There were also videos and cassettes for sale in tandem with Cayce's wisdom. A library/research room was available for writers, researchers, A.R.E. members and the public. The store carried all the popular Cayce health care remedies. And there were gemstones for sale that Cayce prescribed in readings as tools to raise the vibrational energy of certain people for their well-being and development of innate psychic abilities. Housed in the building was a 100-seat auditorium for lectures and hands-on workshops, and a kitchen for classes on food preparation and nutrition according to Cayce's recommendations.

Office space will be leased to professionals and businesses that share an affinity with the Center's ideals. Rooms are available to accommodate colonic hydrotherapists, massage therapists, energy healers, artists, medical doctors and chiropractors who specialize in Cayce-style examinations and treatment. Other sources of income to help maintain the Center involve plans to embrace a community of holistic metaphysical experts. They would offer programs on any topic or discipline compatible with Cayce's ideals and the goals of the Houston A.R.E.'s Search For God Council. Programs would include topics on: psychism, healing with touch, transpersonal therapy, meditation, life planning, exercise, auras, sound/music therapy, color therapy, aromatherapy, philosophy, intuitive guidance, astrology, numerology and classes on how to utilize the many remedies recommended by Cayce. The Center will also be offering college level courses from the A.R.E.'s Atlantic University Learning at a Distance Program, studies in massage with staff from the Virginia Beach Cayce/Reilly School of Massotherapy, and psychic development training from the Edgar Cayce Institute for Intuitive Studies.

Jamail believes the Center will attract people opened to and/or educated in Cayce's philosophy of setting a spiritual ideal, meditation, a Cayce-affirmed diet, stress reduction, exercise and a Christ Consciousness discernment. "We need to take responsibility for our physical, intellectual, emotional and spiritual health," Jamail said. The Center is dedicated to educating people on how to be actively accountable for their lives. They offer options for maintaining and reclaiming good health as delineated by Cayce. Jamail is available at the Center on week days, but individuals can use computers on the premises to find readings for particular remedies relating to ailments they wish to treat. He pointed out that soon customers will be able to discuss the use of Cayce products with the Center's health care professionals on the premises. There will also be a referral list of practitioners in Houston who utilize Cayce health care principles. "We will even show people how to intuitively select the right remedies for healing themselves," Jamail told me. The Center is also planning spa weekends so people can come several times a year to "...vastly improve their health." A spa package would include: massage, group meditation, fume baths, colonics, exercise, lectures and hands-on workshops in sync with Cayce's readings. "We would offer the Meridian Institute's computerized Cayce-style health evaluation, too."

The Meridian Institute is the scientific research team at A.R.E., Virginia Beach. They have applied their extensive studies on Cayce's health care readings to assemble 50 protocols and 3000 questionnaires. Facts about symptoms and other medical particulars are filled out on the survey by a person requesting a computerized health reading. The information is then fed into the computer data base. Details are sorted out by the computer, which matches symptoms to remedies that rejuvenate the body in tandem with Cayce health care. Also included in the Meridian Institute's protocol is an electronic blood count analysis, a check up of the electromagnetic field of the body and an examination of the electrical energy of the meridians. Information from these electronic tests reveals computerized health care wisdom similar to what Cayce would have conveyed if he were doing an actual reading. "We foresee that our Center, and all A.R.E. Centers throughout the world, will eventually use the Meridian Institute's protocol," Jamail explained.

I was interested in exploring some of the approximately 110 popular Cayce remedies stocked on the Center's store shelves. Jamail told me about several of them beginning with Castor Oil. Cayce recommended Castor Oil for various purposes in at least 600 readings. I told him about an article that I recently read concerning researchers at the University of Kansas who discovered an ingredient in the castor bean that retards most skin cancers. "A.R.E. members are familiar with the healing power of Castor Oil through 80 years of use," Jamail stated matter-of-factly. "I could relate thousands of success stories about the curative powers of Castor Oil." As an example, he told me about his brother's triumph over Infectious Hepatitis with the use of Castor Oil packs. Jamail's brother, a Houston Roman Catholic Priest, became infected with the disease after undergoing minor surgery in the 60s. He returned to the hospital repeatedly for conventional treatment, which afforded him no relief. His doctors prescribed a liver transplant, putting him on top of the surgery list because of his status with the Catholic Church. Not wanting to suffer the ordeal of this medical procedure, his brother, who never reconciled Jamail's involvement with what he considered "Cayce's occult philosophies", asked Jamail if Cayce had anything to say about the liver. Jamail told him about the readings for healing the liver and recommended that his brother try Cayce's prescriptions. His brother agreed. Jamail placed a Castor Oil pack over his brother's liver and solar plexus, roughly on the navel and around the right side where there is a high concentration of nerves and organs. A Castor Oil pack in this position reaches the liver and one kidney. The pack was covered with plastic. A heating pad, set for comfort on medium, was placed over the pack which remained in position for an hour-and-a-half. This procedure was repeated once a day. Jamail's brother also took massive doses of vitamin C. "Within 2 weeks, my brother's liver was functioning normally, and to this day he has never had any more trouble with it," stated Jamail.

Cayce saw the combination of 3 to 4 thickness' of white wool unbleached flannel soaked with cold-pressed Castor Oil and applied to the solar plexus as an effective vibrational healing tool. This process facilitates nervous activity so the body functions with proper nerve coordination and is able to better identify how to combat existing health problems. Cold-pressed Castor Oil pressed out of the castor bean is not the kind of Castor Oil bought in drug stores. Drug store Castor Oil has been processed using a heat method to destroy inherent poison in the castor bean. The castor plant is poisonous, and Cayce rarely recommended that it be taken internally. Jamail said that it was the poison of choice for assassination by the Bulgarian KGB during the Cold War. "Today, doctors agree with Cayce about the solar plexus being like a second brain.," Jamail explained. "They now recognize what Cayce stated long ago, that Pyors Patches, which are situated in the solar plexus area, are responsible for triggering the immune system."

He also told me about Mike, an AIDS patient who was helped with the use of Castor Oil packs. A course of treatment was mapped out for Mike by Dr. William McGarey, the Director of the A.R.E. hospital, Phoenix, Arizona. Castor Oil packs were applied to Mike's solar plexus once in the morning and again in the afternoon for an hour, because treatment once a day was not effective for him. "Mike had a very bad case of AIDS," Jamail explained. "He had lost a lot of weight, looked emaciated, and developed opportunistic infections, which is what AIDS patients usually die from." The task was to trigger the chemical in Mike's body that would create an alkaline environment which is necessary for avoiding infection. Jamail advised Mike to change his diet to 90% alkaline foods consisting mainly of vegetables, raw and lightly cooked. Mike also began a regimen of meditation, stress reduction and exercise. "For about a year, Mike's 'T" cell count had alarmingly dropped, but within 28 days of the Castor Oil pack treatments and an alkaline diet, his "T" cell count rebounded to a healthy 109," Jamail stated. Within 2 months, Mike began gaining weight and he felt good enough to look for a job.

Jamail asked me if I had read Discover Magazine's, October, 1996, feature on how "T" cells fight health problems in the body. In the case of cancer, however, "T" cells help augment its growth through the release of an enzyme. The article, Jamail said, explained that scientists were working to find a solution on how to turn the "T" cell off so it would stop the advancement of cancer's growth. "Cayce gave us the answer more than 80 years ago when he talked about alkalizing the system with a diet of 80% primarily raw vegetables and salads, fish, poultry and very little meat."

Once a month, 3 nights in a row, Jamail uses a Castor Oil pack on himself for nerve coordination. While using the pack, he reads an inspirational book to bring spirit, attitude and emotion into the healing process while imagining his body flowing with harmonious healing vibrations. The Castor Oil pack stays in place for about an hour-and-a-half. "If I were ill, I would do it every day, and I might actually see toxins pulled out of my body staining the pack with dark spots," he explained. Placement of the pack, length of time it remains on the body and number of times the procedure is repeated each day varies according to the ailment being treated. Soiled white flannel can be washed and reused for a few times before discarding it. After using the pack, baking soda should be massaged over the treated area to absorb toxins, and then immediately rinsed off so the toxins do not go back into the body. Evening is the best time to apply a pack because that is when most people are restful and have fewer interruptions. But if this is not possible, anytime will do.

I asked him about Glyco-Thymoline, another product on the store shelf that Cayce frequently spoke about in readings. He tells me that it is an alkaline antiseptic made of Eucalyptol, Menthol, Pine Oil, and Thymol. The manufacturer states that these ingredients are gentle enough to use on a baby's skin. Glyco-Thymoline is a natural mouthwash and gargle. It is also used to alkalize the system when a cold is coming on by taking 8 to10 drops in a glass of warm water, once in the morning and once in the evening. Jamail suggested using Glyco-Thymoline as an eyewash diluted with 2 parts of distilled water to 1 part Glyco-Thymoline. He told me that several years ago his eyes would not stop tearing, but that his optometrist did not know the cause. The optometrist thought that living in an urban environment caused all kinds of unknown irritants to infect the eyes and the body. "He prescribed drops for $60 that did not help my eyes," Jamail told me. When he consulted Cayce's readings for a remedy, he found that Glyco-Thymoline was suggested as an eye wash. Within 5 days of using the solution, the tearing stopped and his eyes completely cleared up.

"What is Ipsab?" I asked Jamail, pointing to a package on the shelf. He told me that Ipsab is a tooth powder and gum massager and that there are other Ipsab related remedies for oral hygiene recommended in Cayce's readings. The major ingredients in Ipsab are prickly ash bark and iodine. "American Indians used Ipsab as toothache medicine. It used to be the main ingredient of Ipana toothpaste," Jamail says. "For alleviating gum problems, make a watery solution of the powder and massage it onto the gums."

I also questioned Jamail about Calcios, a Cayce prescribed calcium supplement. He informs me that most store brand calcium supplements are based on oyster shell or a similar derivative. But Calcios, a spreadable paste, is made of bone with pancreatin, pepsin and hydrochloric acid, along with other trace minerals, including iodine. "It is so potent that only a small amount consumed on one cracker wafer 3 times a week supplies 328 milligrams of calcium," Jamail said. "Cayce's readings explained that it was rapidly and easily assimilated and immediately used where it is needed in the body." Jamail took Calcios while recovering from injuries sustained when he was mugged. The assault shattered his left side, broke his collar bone, ribs and shoulder blades, fracturing and stressing his joints. "I was in my 50s, and my physical therapist and MD were amazed because my bones healed so fast. It was Calcios that helped me do it," Jamail maintained.

The store also carries Animated Ash and Carbon Ash, which Cayce recommended for oxygenating the body. Jamail told me that recently, two Rice University chemists, Rick Smalley and Robert Curl, received Nobel Prizes for their discovery of Carbon 60, a molecule of carbon shaped like a soccer ball. They named it Buckminster Fullerine after Buckminster Fuller, the architect of the geodesic dome. At first, doctors didn't know what to do with the "new" discovery. But researchers recently came to the conclusion that the Carbon 60 element can carry drugs used to treat various ills. "Cayce's readings stated that Carbon Ash carries oxygen which can destroy cancer cells, a fact that the A.R.E. has known and utilized for over 80 years," Jamail said, smiling.

Charred Oak Keg with 100% Apple Brandy is another popular Cayce remedy. "It is ordered most often for people with severe respiratory problems," explained Jamail. Cayce recommended it for treatment of TB and it is very effective in treating emphysema. One of the success stories Jamail related is about a 100-year-old man suffering from emphysema. He was able to discontinue his oxygen treatments with the use of Charred Oak Keg with 100% Apple Brandy.

I scanned the array of Cayce remedies and Cayce-related products stocked in the store: cola syrup for alkalizing the body, various tonics, creams, oils, pastes, ointments, compounds, moisturizers, salves, tablets, powers, herbal extracts, laxatives, herbal deodorant, herbal supplements, antacids, lip balm, natural sedatives like Lithia Water and Valerian Tincture, rubbing alcohol, syrups, vitamins, aromatherapy oils, minerals, soaps, shampoos, copper magnetic bracelets, digestive enzymes, fungacides, hemorrhoid astringent, antiseptics and various Cayce advocated apparatuses for a variety of conditions. Also in the offering were foods that Cayce spoke of: Steel Cut Oats, Fig Syrup, Mullein Leaves for tea, olive oil, garlic oil, Beet Sugar and raw almonds. Cayce described Beet Sugar as a natural sweetener that would not strain the system like sugar in any other form. He recommended raw almonds as an excellent source of protein, vitamins, minerals, essential fatty acids calcium, iron, potassium, phosphorus and trace minerals like zinc and copper. In reading 3180-3 he said: ***"A person who eats two or three almonds each day need never fear cancer."***

A color therapy kit with colored gels and a lamp to utilize them caught my eye. "Cayce said that if we learn how to use color it would be as effective as pharmaceuticals," Jamail told me. "But he never went into what that meant or how to do it. However, last year a 93-year old woman who had been an A.R.E. member since the mid 30s donated her book collection to us. It included *Let There Be Light*, a book about the healing power of color by Darius Denshah."

Denshah lived during the first half of the century and died in '65. The Denshah Society, which is still in existence, provides information on color therapy. Carl Bohannon, the Center Complex's Co-Director, read Denshah's book and ordered a set of theatrical colored gels from the Denshah Society. He put together a kit for himself right before he came down with a nasty strain of the flu. Following the instructions that came with the gels for treatment of flu, stuffed sinuses and head-colds, Bohannon sat in a dark room and exposed the trunk of his body for one hour to the green gel reflected with the lamp. Then he used a tangerine color, for the same length of time, focused on the upper portion of his body. He did not notice any physical change with the green color, but within 10 minutes of using the tangerine, he felt and heard his sinuses pop open as they drained. For 3 days Bohannon's head remained clear and he no longer had a headache. When the symptoms returned, he repeated the color therapy again, only this time it was even more effective, and his flu vanished.

Cayce saw the endocrine glands and their related chakra frequencies as potent vehicles of control over body functions. Bohannon experimented with colored light frequencies on various chakras. Applying what he learned about how color interacts electromagnetically with the body's chakra energy fields to influence the rebalancing of the system, Bohannon created a color kit with a lamp and 11 colored gels. He offered workshops through the A.R.E. to demonstrate the power of color. A purple color was applied on someone in the audience who was having a severe migraine headache. "You could see in her eyes that she was in a lot of pain, and in her case she lost sight in her right eye every time a migraine struck her," Bohannon said. The woman sat under a purple light for 20 minutes, and her migraine disappeared as the vision in her right eye returned. "We kept in touch, and she told us that she continued to treat herself with the purple color which prevented a migraine from developing."

I asked about the Violet Ray, a popular appliance recommended by Cayce in over 800 readings. It has a high voltage output of approximately 50,000 volts, and a frequency of over one-million cycles per second. When it is turned on, the color of the gas in the bulb appears violet, which is how the device got its name. Chiropractors, massage therapists and hairdressers implement it to stimulate glands, local circulation and nerve coordination. The Violet Ray has, among other things, improved vision, alleviated anemia and arthritis and stopped hair loss.

"Who manufactures the Cayce remedies?" I asked. Jamail told me that there are two companies that produce the products: the Heritage Store, Virginia Beach, and Baar Products, Pennsylvania. Bruce Baar formerly worked for Johnson & Johnson and has an agreement with the A.R.E., which closely supervises his methods of production. "Cayce was very particular about how the remedies were combined," Jamail explained. "He gave specific instructions on how and when to add certain ingredients in order to get a particular chemical reaction." It was Cayce's intent that the remedy be taken immediately after it was formulated for maximum effectiveness. Years ago this was possible because the local pharmacy would prepare the mixture while you waited. But today, the only way this could be expedited would be to teach people to make the remedies themselves. "We plan to do that when we have an herbalist/naturopath on the premises," Jamail said. Another long range Center plan is to grow herbs and vegetables on the premises or nearby, in order to get the full nutritional vibrational benefit that our bodies require. Cayce said that shipped herbs and foods from across the country reduce or nullify their value.

"That's a Wet-Cell Battery!" I said, recognizing a large cylindrical jar. The lid on the jar had 2 holes in it for copper and nickel poles and plates, battery solution chemicals and lead wires. Cayce mentioned the Wet-Cell in over 900 readings to help the nervous system by supplying life force vibrations to the body. Jamail explained that the body is like a battery. It produces its own electricity, which can become unbalanced or depleted with injury or disease. The Wet-Cell Battery is comparable to a booster cable, producing needed electrical energy, via its connection to the body, to get the healing and regenerating process started with no side effects or pain. There is a choice of six different solutions to place in the jar: gold chloride, silver nitrate, tincture of iron, camphor spirits, atomidine and Glyco-Thymoline. They are implemented homeopathically by introducing vibrations of the mineral into the body, which responds as if the actual whole mineral has been ingested, but without the toxic side effects. Jamail said that gold chloride administered through the Wet-Cell Battery solution jar, and an alkaline diet, can relieve arthritis. This is what Cayce said in the 20s. Cayce also suggested that by using the gold and silver mineral solution in the Wet-Cell Battery solution jar, we could regenerate nerves, brain cells and other parts of the body. "Up until a few months ago, science disagreed with Cayce. But now scientists are saying that brain cells and nerve cells can reproduce and repair themselves, given the proper stimulus and nutrition," Jamail said.

The wires for the Wet-Cell Battery are connected to different parts of the body depending on what is being treated. Information about connections to appropriate places on the body is in the Cayce readings. It is also contained in the book *The Radial Appliance and Wet-Cell Battery, Two Electrotherapeutic Devices Recommended By Edgar Cayce*, written by David McMillan, MA and Douglas G. Richards, Ph.D., Lifeline Press, Virginia Beach, Virginia. For treatment of a specific illness, like Multiple Sclerosis, a detailed protocol is available from the Meridian Institute, Virginia Beach. "Controlling MS with the Cayce approach, which includes the Wet-Cell Battery, has been very successful," Jamail pointed out. He knew of a man in Virginia Beach who lectures about his recovery from ALS using the Wet-Cell battery. But he is the only person Jamail knows of who recovered from ALS using the Cayce approach. "I believe that's because it takes a lot of patience to use the Wet-Cell Battery several hours a day. It requires someone to work with you, since treatment is done in multiple applications with massage." Jamail explained. "It took him 18 months to go from being totally bedridden to becoming ambulatory and functioning again."

Another device stocked by the Center's store is the Radial Appliance, recommended in over 400 readings by Cayce. It is made to Cayce's specifications: two pieces of carbon 60 steel, sandwiched together with glass, surrounded by carbon and encased in a square box. The Radial Appliance comes with lead wire electrodes to attach to the body, nickel plates, a solution jar and mineral solutions. Subtle vibrations of gold, silver and iron can be introduced to the solution jar to generate needed red blood cells for anemics. The Radial Appliance is helpful for many other conditions including insomnia rooted in mental strain that has caused the upper lobe of the brain to overload with energy so it difficult to relax and sleep. "Sometimes, walking around will help balance the energy, but for me, the Radial Appliance is like a switch that deeply relaxes me so I can fall asleep instantly," said Carl Bohannon, Co-Director of the Center Complex, who joined us on the tour. Bohannon told me that 30 minutes before use, the appliance should be placed in a bucket of ice until it gets down below 40 degrees. This is the necessary temperature to balance the body's energy. The Radial Appliance got its name because it is used in a radial pattern. One electrode is attached on the right wrist and one on the left ankle. The electrodes are then rotated to the left wrist and the right ankle, followed by the electrodes being attached to the left ankle and the right wrist. This rotation is continued systematically, generally for an hour at a time, until you begin to relax.

Each person has a distinct energetic magnetism. The energy frequency emitted contains the vibration of what we do and believe, the general condition of the body, and everything else about us. These signals are picked up and recorded in the matrix of the steel, which is the reason Cayce said to use the Radial Appliance only when in a positive frame of mind. Otherwise, the device will record anger or any negativity in you and then feed it back to you.

Bohannon explained that even the person who assembles the Radial Appliance should be in a prayerful attitude while building it. The device will pick up vibrations of whatever that person is thinking or doing at the time of assembly, and return them to whoever uses the appliance. He cited an example in which Cayce had advised the use of the Radial Appliance in a reading for a particular woman. The man who built the appliance for her had a fight with his wife and was very angry when he went to his garage to construct the apparatus. A month later the woman returned to Cayce complaining that she was angry all the time. Cayce did another reading for her and saw that the man who built the Radial Appliance had passed his anger to her via the device that he built. He also told the builder of the Radial Appliance that he had karma to face because of his disregard for the warning not to build an appliance while in a state of anger.

"You should never drink alcohol while using the Radial Appliance, because it could build a pattern of alcohol dependency in the body," Bohannon cautioned. It is always necessary to be in a prayerful, uplifting frame of mind while using it. After 30 days of everyday use, the appliance will have retained enough of your positive vibrational energy. If you are feeling depressed or have a negative attitude, you can reconnect the appliance to your body, and it will immediately reenergize you with your positive vibrations which it has retained. "Everyone should meditate with the Radial Appliance because it makes the meditation more powerful," Bohannon recommended. He reminded me that Cayce said the most powerful thing you can do is to set up a spiritual ideal.

Bohannon suggested focusing on your spiritual ideal before you use a brand new Radial Appliance because it will feed your ideal back to you each time you use the appliance.

The Radial Appliance was initially priced at approximately $200. Then they made a simpler version of it, like the one used at the A.R.E. hospital in the 20s. Over a period of 15 years it has been updated many times with more durable, affordable, modern material. Each version of the Radial Appliance has always been assessed by a psychic. The only specifications that remain constant are the kind of steel Cayce specified and that the appliance be packed in charcoal and cooled down for use. The current cost is at an all-time low of $55, and a psychic determined that the appliance is 90% as effective as the expensive version. "A lower price makes it affordable for more people," said Jamail. "Using any version is 100% better than not using it at all."

"Why doesn't every medical doctor know about and utilize the Radial Appliance for patients, as well as other Cayce devices and products?" I asked. "Conventional medical science is just finding out about the use of subtle energy," Jamail explained. At the A.R.E. Meridian Institute, medical doctors, scientists and researchers are doing continuing trials with Cayce's approach on various ailments. Jamail told me that the Meridian Institute is writing and publishing protocols for a number of the Cayce remedies, and they are being well received. People come to the A.R.E.'s H.R.R.C. (Health & Rejuvenation Research Center) programs and stay for 2 or 3 weeks. They go through a protocol of a strict diet, daily meditation and the whole Cayce holistic regimen. This includes the use of various Cayce recommended appliances and tests that the medical staff administers. "In 3 weeks almost all patients have a remarkable health change for the better," Jamail said. "But when they return home to their old habits, situations, doubts, fears, lack of support and unavailable techniques, they are really frustrated to find that their health reverts back to where they began when they first came to the H.R.R.C."

At the end of my visit to the Houston A.R.E. Center Complex, Bohannon said, "We trust Mr. Cayce's readings, which have been tried and tested, time and again, to prove that he knew what he was talking about." Several years ago, for example, a friend of Bohannon's had a heart attack and was told by his doctors that his arteries were obstructed. Because Bohannon's friend meditates, is a vegetarian, and has a generally healthy lifestyle, he could not understand why he had developed this condition. After consulting the readings, he found that Cayce said that the type of heart condition he had was due to an electrical imbalance between the heart and liver. Cayce gave directions about how to use the Radial Appliance to correct the electrical imbalance. He also recommended alkalizing the body with diet to reverse the condition. Bohannon and Jamail had thought

Cayce missed seeing the connection of cholesterol as the culprit causing the heart condition. But then they read about a new theory in the newspaper concerning arteriosclerosis. It said that medical science now believes the root cause of arteriosclerosis is a low grade bacterial infection inside the walls of the arteries that is responsible for scarring and collecting plaque. Doctors now think the condition is treatable with an antibiotic. "Cayce was saying, balance the energy around the organ and alkalize the system so the body can naturally take care of the invading bacterial agent," Bohannon concluded. "We realized that if it doesn't look like Mr. Cayce's readings are accurate, it's only because we can't "*see*" what he was able to "*see*". Mr. Cayce was always right on target!"

....

Contact Ed Jamail And Carl Bohannon at:

Houston A.R.E. Center,
7800 Amelia, Houston, TX. 77055
Telephone: 713-263-1006 or
Tel/Fax: 713-522-5084
Email: are-houston@worldnet.att.net

....

RECOMMENDED READING

(Available at the Houston A.R.E. Center Complex)

AN EDGAR CAYCE HOME MEDICINE GUIDE
Compiled by the Editors at A.R.E.
(Foreword by Gladys Davis Turner, Edgar Cayce's Secretary)
A.R.E. Press, June, 1992

THE OIL THAT HEALS
William McGarey, MD
A.R.E. Press, 1993

PHYSICIANS REFERENCE NOTEBOOK
William McGarey, MD
A.R.E. Press, 2000

HEALTH THROUGH DRUGLESS THERAPY
Harold Reilly, MD
A.R.E. Press, 1998

KEYS TO HEALTH
Eric Mein, MD
Tom Doherty Associates, 1995

NOURISHING THE BODY TEMPLE:
Edgar Cayce's Approach to Nutrition
Simone Gabbay, R.N.C.P.
A.R.E. Press, 1999

EDGAR CAYCE'S DIET AND RECIPE GUIDE
Compiled by the Editors of the A.R.E. Press, 1999

....

11

MAGNETIC FIELD THERAPY
An Interview With Mary Broeringmeyer, DC

....

Let both prongs of the magnet touch the body;
not rubbed, though, as to cause irritation,
but held upward, so as to demagnetize at each center.

EDGAR CAYCE
Reading 2820-1 (21) for a 52 year old male
suffering from severe headaches, a choking sensation
in the throat and other symptoms, 1942

The late **Mary Broeringmeyer, DC** graduated from Logan Chiropractic College in St. Louis, Missouri. While married to her first husband, an Osteopath and surgeon, she served as his assistant and office manager. She shared his interest in nutrition and natural health remedies which lead her to pursue a career in natural health care. After his death, she entered Logan Chiropractic College where she met Dr. Richard Broeringmeyer, who became her second husband. They conducted a successful Chiropractic and nutritional practice in Murray, Kentucky, while Dr. Richard Broeringmeyer was engaged in research and development of biomagnetic energies for measuring and treating body imbalances. The Broeringmeyer's co-partnered Health Industries, Inc., Murray, Kentucky, a bio-magnetic firm.

The conditions here may be best retarded by the use at times, about once a week, of a magnet of sufficient strength to raise a railroad spike - this being passed over affected areas, see? This will aid in demagnetizing or producing a vibration that will destroy the active forces of the consuming of cells being enlivened by the infection itself.

EDGAR CAYCE
Reading 3313-1 (4)
For a 58 year old female
suffering from throat cancer, 1943

....

The late **Richard Broeringmeyer, PhD, DC, ND** authored eight books on natural health including *Principles of Magnetic Therapy, Colon Therapy Manual* and *Nutritionally Speaking.* He spent many years gathering information for the International Biomagnetic Association on the affects of magnets on cells, organs and the various systems of the body. Dr. Broeringmeyer trained doctors and health care professionals on the proper application of magnets. He was a member of the American Chiropractic Association, Council of Nutrition, International Academy of Preventive Medicine, the American Nutrition Society, International College of Physicians and Surgeons (Homeopathic), and the Maryland Homeopathic Medical Society. Dr. Broeringmeyer was the president of Health Industries, Inc., Murray, Kentucky.

MAGNETIC FIELD THERAPY
An Interview With Mary Broeringmeyer, DC

I first became aware of using magnets to alleviate pain in readings done by Edgar Cayce in the 1940s, a time when therapeutic magnets weren't even in existence. Nevertheless, in several readings, Cayce prescribed Magnetic Field Therapy, describing the preparation of the magnet to help alleviate illness and pain. In reading 569-28 (5) given in 1943 for a 62 year old female suffering from abdominal cancer, Cayce said, ***"There might be had some aid in relief if there would be prepared in the present a very strong magnet, this encased in metal - as in German Silver - and this applied over the area in the abdomen where there are those great pains..."***

Restoring health to the body with a magnet seemed like sorcerer's magic in a fairy tale. Still, I toyed with the idea of ridding myself of sporadic lower back pain with a therapeutic magnet. I called a company listed under "Magnets" in the Yellow Pages, but they sold only industrial magnets. They suggested that I phone Health Industries, Inc., a company in Kentucky that manufactured magnetic products for health enhancement. The owner, Mary Broeringmeyer, a Chiropractor, educated me about biomagnets and the magnetic nature of cells in the body.

Dr. Broeringmeyer told me that electrolytic salts exist in the blood stream, generating electric currents associated with natural magnetic fields of varying strengths. In 1954, the Nobel Prize was awarded to Dr. Linus Pauling for his discovery of magnetic fields in hemoglobin (protein coloring matter of the red blood corpuscles), which convey oxygen to the tissues. Basically, tiny magnetic cells are the fundamental constituents of all body organs. Every organ produces its own magnetic field, fluctuating according to activity, rest, nutrition and other external influences. Disturbances occurring in the balance of an organ's magnetic field throw off its normal functioning, resulting in a mild or serious ailment, depending on the importance of the organ affected. Magnetic Field Therapy helps adjust the equilibrium of the body's electrical pattern for maximum health.

A treating magnet placed on an ailing part of the body, attracts and moves electrically charged particles in the blood stream. But the magnetic field produced by the magnet is only a secondary energy field moving the highly charged particles. No energy passes from the magnetic field of the magnet into the person. The energy involved is the spinning of electrons already present. A healthy cell spins counterclockwise while its nucleus spins clockwise; a diseased cell spins clockwise while its nucleus spins counterclockwise. Healthy cells give off energy; diseased cells draw energy from the body to the disease. Reversing the spin of the diseased cell maintains energy and helps the body fight illness. "Magnetic Therapy is very useful for reversing the spin of a diseased cell and creating an optimum environment for the body to heal itself of a multitude of ailments," Broeringmeyer said. (See: *Maladies Benefited By Magnetic Therapy*, at end of chapter). As the cells spin, blood vessels dilate implementing greater blood flow. This, in turn, promotes oxygen-carrying capacity enabling nutrient-rich blood to circulate around the treated area. "Better circulation is fundamental to good health, boosting the energy necessary to rapidly detoxify the body of wastes," Broeringmeyer explained. "This process is essential to the body's innate capacity to heal itself."

"Can a magnet relieve lower back pain?" I asked. Broeringmeyer said she had success using Magnetic Field Therapy on many patients suffering from back pain. However, she cautioned that using a magnet was not always a substitute for medical treatment. "Magnetic Field Therapy is often best used in conjunction with a dietary, chemical, manipulative or physical therapy program," she said.

Some scientists believe that much of chronic back, neck, shoulder and chest pain, inflammation, stiffness, spasm, chronic fatigue, listlessness, insomnia, nervousness, stress and tumors are a direct result of our electronic environment overwhelming the earth's natural magnetic field. Continual electromagnetic bombardment from home appliances, televisions, computers, alarm clocks, steel frame and structured buildings, cars, electric trains, planes and ships absorbing a large portion of the magnetic lines of the earth's magnetic field, are elements contributing to hazardous or harmful affects on the human body. Broeringmeyer believes that another factor associated with many ailments is a 50% decrease in the strength of the earth's magnetic field. "This phenomena has gradually taken place over the last 500 years along with shifts in the angles of the earth's magnetic field," she said. Her late husband, Dr. Richard Broeringmeyer, a recognized authority on biomagnets, thought it was possible to eliminate the detrimental affects of electromagnetic fields. His treatment entailed exposing the body to high strength magnets totaling 4200 gauss, for 10 minutes in the morning and 10 minutes at night. Magnets range in strength from 500 to 5000 gauss field intensity, and super magnets used for cancer research programs are 12,500 gauss.

I purchased a 4 by 5 inch magnetic "pain pad" that Broeringmeyer suggested for treatment of lower back pain. It was made of a special rubber compound and contained a high content of barium ferrite to which a permanent magnetic structure was added. Broeringmeyer said to tape the pad to the body, directly over the aching area, with the negative "north-seeking" side on the body. She explained the semantics of "north-seeking" and "south-seeking": "north-seeking" and "north" are terms often mistakenly used interchangeably; the same holds true for "south-seeking" and "south". Originally, the navigator called the compass needle pointing to the North Pole of the earth, "north pole" and the compass needle pointing to the South Pole of the earth "south pole". This is incorrect, because like poles repel and opposite poles attract. The compass needle pointing to the true physical North Pole of the earth, more accurately known as "north-seeking", is actually south pole. And the compass needle pointing to the true physical South Pole of the earth, more accurately known as "south-seeking", is actually north pole. The Encyclopedia Britannica recognizes this semantic confusion and recommends using the electrical terms "positive" and "negative" rather than "north pole" and "south pole", because magnetic poles and electric poles are the same in terms of the magnetism present. It is important to understand the difference between the conventional and corrected way of naming north and south magnetic polarity, because some manufacturers of therapeutic magnets still use the incorrect definition. "This semantic confusion can cause inappropriate use of biomagnetic products," she said.

"Does Magnetic Field Therapy have side effects?" I asked.

"Based on my experience, I know that the proper application of the negative, north-seeking end of the magnet, in the correct gauss strength, can be effective and safely used 24-hours a day with no side effects," she told me. However, Broeringmeyer recommended cautious use of magnets for people with programmed implants such as pacemakers. Pregnant women are advised not to use bio-magnets because there is not enough data on the application of Magnetic Field Therapy during pregnancy. A waiting period of 90 minutes after eating a meal is suggested before placing a magnet on the abdomen to prevent interference with the digestive process. "The positive, south-seeking side of a magnet should be used prudently," Dr. Broeringmeyer advised. "Allegedly it can have harmful affects such as: risk of seizures, hallucinations, insomnia, hyperactivity, stimulation of bacteria, tumors and addictive behavior." *(See end of chapter for list of characteristic responses to positive (south-seeking) and negative (north-seeking) magnetic fields.)*

When the "pain-pad" arrived in the mail, I taped the clearly marked, negative (north-seeking) side of the flexible pad directly to my skin, over the ache in my lower back. It remained in place continuously for one day. I immediately experienced some relief, and my lower back pain disappeared completely in less than 24-hours. My back remained in stable condition after removing the "pain-pad".

In the package with the "pain-pad" was a copy of *Principles of Magnetic Therapy*, a book written by Dr. Richard Broeringmeyer. One of the chapters discussed the work of American scientists Albert Roy David and Walter C. Rawls, Jr. In the 1970s, David and Rawls achieved a 90% success rate in curing cancer implanted on the skin of rodents, using Magnetic Field Therapy. However, their work was not acknowledged in peer-reviewed medical literature until 20 years after their accomplishments. In September, 1990, the *Journal of the National Medical Association* published their diagram clearly showing that the growth of lung carcinoma cells were inhibited when placed within a negative magnetic field.

"Most conventional doctors in the USA do not use therapeutic magnets to treat patients," Dr. Richard Broeringmeyer explained. Nevertheless, they routinely use the application of magnetism for diagnostic purposes: magnetoencephalograms to record brain waves, magnetic resonance imaging for detailed images of internal body parts and magnetic coils in wraps to penetrate and facilitate mending of bone breaks resistant to healing.

In Japan, magnets are sold in pharmacies over-the-counter as government approved medical devices. Many physicians in European and Asian hospitals routinely use therapeutic magnets as an accepted method of treatment. Millions of people in the USA, Asia, Europe and Canada use Magnetic Field Therapy for healing, because biomagnets work rapidly and are non-invasive, non-toxic, inexpensive, simple to use and have no adverse side effects when utilized properly. It is currently illegal in the USA to sell a magnet as a medical device. Restrictions do not apply on magnets under 1000 gauss that are sold for self-help purposes. It was Dr. Richard Broeringmeyer's belief that one of the reasons Magnetic Field Therapy has been put on the back burner in the USA is because commercial enterprise can not profit from it like it does from antibiotics, costly medications, patent tablets and capsules, and injections professed to afford quick relief.

Since experiencing the "pain-pad", I have tried other therapeutic magnets when aches and pains have cropped up. I found that Broeringmeyer's line of round, coin-sized, hard disc magnets fitted comfortably on my wrists, knees and small areas of my body. Also, I have attended seminars sponsored by other companies that manufacture biomagnetic products. Some specialize in therapeutic magnets of alternate polarity, with north and south magnetic poles on the same flat surface, in a variety of configurations. They use the traditional method for naming the poles. Alternate polarity patterning is believed to mathematically increase the probability that blood vessels, at any angle and position in the body, will cross the magnetic field in the magnetic pad. Product lines include an impressive array of items ranging in price from approximately $5 to $2,500.

One of the more costly items is a magnetic mattress constructed with over 100 magnets, each with a strength of 800 gauss. The mattress is said to encourage peaceful sleep and more energy. However, I learned that gauss strength is not the key variable influencing effectiveness of other biogmagnetic products, because the force of the magnetic field varies inversely with the square of the distance. This is particularly important when evaluating magnetic mattresses and pillows, because the distance from the target area is subject to constant fluctuation.

There are many alternate polarity biomagnetic products that I would like to try. One of them is a quilt designed to reflect body heat back into the body, changing the pH which reduces acidity; and there is a car seat pad made of rubberthane that the manufacturer says keeps the body generally comfortable by disbursing body moisture. "A Chiropractor On A Stick" is the nickname for a magnetic alternate polarity rolling pin meant to be wheeled up and down the back. It is said that a half-hour rollout simulates a night of sleep. Another biomagnetic product on my "wish list" is a pair of alternate polarity magnetic cylinders on a handle designed to penetrate cartilage, soft tissue and hard tissue up to 18 inches. Ultra sound and deep heat used by Chiropractors and medical doctors only penetrates the skin 3/8 of an inch. And I want to try a magnetic face mask made with small inserted circular magnets of alternate polarity. The mask, worn a few hours at night, is designed to encourage movement of healthier cells to the surface of the skin. Noted results are a decrease in wrinkles, lines, dark circles, puffy eyes and improvement in skin texture. Biomagnetic headboards are also available. They are assembled with four large, evenly spaced ceramic magnets held in place along a metal strip running across the front of the headboard. The magnets are used on the negative (north-seeking) side about an inch or two away from the head. Biomagnetic headboards are meant to promote the production of melatonin, which encourages relaxation and a good night's sleep.

And last, but certainly not least, are magnetic innersoles that many biomagnetic companies offer. Some have alternate polarity, while other styles have a negative (north-seeking) side and a positive (south-seeking) side. The negative (north-seeking) side is placed against the soles of the feet. Magnetic innersoles are said to increase strength up to 20-percent, from the bottom of the feet to the tips of the hands. Knight-Ridder Newspapers published a story on May 31, 1997 about pro golfers who have gotten quick and continuous relief from significant back, arm and leg pain by wearing magnetic innersoles and other biomagnetic products. As a result of this, they have come out of retirement to play in golf tournaments, pain free, winning top dollars.

I purchased a pair of magnetic innersoles for my mother who is often confined to bed with arthritic pain. At first she did not want to try the innersoles, because she believed it was some sort of hoax. Her rigid attitude quickly changed when she took a chance and discovered that wearing the innersoles substantially relieved her arthritic pain, and increased her energy so she was able to get back on her feet. My mother and I now know that restoring health with the aid of a therapeutic magnet is not a sorcerer's magic. Forgive us, Mr. Cayce! Good health, as explained in the readings, is the sum total of electromagnetic balance, what we eat, drink, breathe, think and feel.

I have had wonderful success treating patients with therapeutic magnets for sprains, strains, broken bones, cuts, joint conditions and circulatory disorders. It should be made clear that magnets do not heal anything, they only stimulate the body's capacity to heal itself.

David M. Redding, DC
Friendswood, TX

MALADIES BENEFITED BY MAGNETIC FIELD THERAPY

Documented case studies from reputable medical journal studies by scientists and medical doctors have reported benefits of biomagnetic therapy for:

* Acute injuries
* Migraine Headaches
* Insomnia
* Sinus Congestion
* High and Low blood Sugar
* Infection
* Dizziness
* Loss of Motor function
* Sunburn
* Motion Sickness
* Wrinkles
* Colitis
* Intestinal Parasites
* Liver Disorders
* Nervousness
* Diabetes Mellitus
* Adrenal Gland Imbalance
* Hiatus Hernia of Diaphragm
* Liver Disease
* Gall Bladder Disease
* Pancreatic Disease
* Stomach Dysfunction and Ulcers
* Intestinal Disorders
* Diverticulitis
* Kidney Disease
* Menstrual Irregularity
* Prostrate Problems
* Bladder Weakness
* Spleen Malfunction
* Eating Disorders
* Addictions
* Thyroid Malfunction
* Cataracts
* Glaucoma

* Alzheimer's Disease
* Cerebral Palsy
* Schizophrenia
* Depression
* TMJ
* Cancer, and many other ailments

ACTIONS OF NEGATIVE (NORTH) POLE MAGNETIC ENERGY

* Sedates, giving a calming, recuperative effect.

* Lessens or completely arrests pain due to hyperactivity, 3rd degree burns, nerve pain, infections caused by inflammation, trauma, or environment.

* Increases alkalinity, to the point of pH normalization (acid/alkaline) of various body fluids out of balance due to illness or abnormal conditions, never producing an over alkalinized condition.

* Vasoconstricts and contracts.

* Draws fluid.

* Arrests protein activity.

* Controls wound bleeding and minor hemorrhage.

* Increases potassium ions, decreases hydrogen ion concentration, and decreases abnormal inorganic calcium ions.

* Dissolves fatty material, calcium deposits around arthritic joints, reduces arthritic inflammation in general, and can reduce cholesterol buildup on inner walls of the veins and arteries.

* Increases mental alertness.

* Increases tissue oxygen to all affected tissues
  but never produces
  oxidized free radicals.

* Slows multiplication of microorganisms; fights infections by the replication of microorganisms and destruction of pathogenic bacteria.

* Attracts white and red blood cells to aid healing.

* Slows heart rate.

* Decreases hydrogen and increases oxygen causing an alkaline metabolic reaction that brings the organ or tissue back to normal.

* Slows down metabolic processes and can extend life span.

* Shrinks tumor and arrests cancer.

ACTIONS OF POSITIVE (SOUTH POLE) MAGNETIC ENERGY

* Activating energy.

* Can increase pain.

* Reduces alkaline state in system, cells, or organs, and can be used to change an alkaline bladder or its normal acid level.

* Enlarges, expands, makes more pliable, and increases the flow of all body fluids by reducing tension and constriction with no weakening of veins, arteries, or capillaries.

* Increases fluids by softening and expanding the capillary canals thereby making possible a greater flow of circulation of all body fluids.

* Softens hardened capillary canals and hardened arteries, and makes organs and tissues flexible.

* Opens canals by expanding and softening the walls of the problem areas.

* Assists in the production of red cells especially where there is a condition that normally would limit or reduce the production of the red cells.

* Improves digestion by increasing acid levels which break down the food for better absorption.

* Increases protein activity enhancing all cellular matter not affected by disease or complaint.

* Increases heartbeat and stimulates organ function.

* Can irritate tissue.

* Speeds metabolic processes.

* Increases sodium. Potassium must predominate in the cells; sodium must predominate in the blood and serum or chronic disease begins.

* Decreases oxygenation of tissue and can block the detoxifying process.

* Can increase the hydrogen ion and create a magnetic field which can normalize the pH of a tissue or organ when it is unbalanced and hypo functioning.

* Can disorganize the central nervous system with overexposure.

Speeds up multiplication of microorganisms such as viruses and bacteria with overexposure. (***DO NOT TREAT TUMORS, CANCEROUS CONDITIONS, OR INFECTIONS WITH THE BIOMAGNETIC SOUTH POLE FIELDS.)***

For further information about Biomagnetics contact:

Health Industries, Inc.
4745 State Route 94 East
Murray, KY 42071
1-800-626-3386

Medical Magnetics of Houston
PO Box 2941
Spring, TX 77383
281-367-6168

Magnetherapy, Inc.
Tec Tonic Management
950 North Congress Avenue
Revera Beach, FL 33404-6400
561-882-0092

RECOMMENDED READING

DISCOVERY OF MAGNETIC HEALTH
George J. Washnis and Richard Z. Hricak
NOVA Publishing Company, 1993

THE BODY ELECTRIC
Robert O. Becker, MD
William Morrow & Co., NY, 1998

Also to quiet the nagging pains at times there may be used a very heavy magnet over the areas where the distresses are indicated. Hold this very close, or upon the flesh of the body - it will, as it were, demagnetize the energies producing the irritation to the body...

EDGAR CAYCE
Reading 3219-1 (11)

12

MASSAGE:
Like Medicine for the Body, Mind, and Spirit
An Interview With: Francis B. Sporer, MA, AMTA, NCTMB, CMT-VA

....

Massage applications are excellent for each body.

EDGAR CAYCE
Reading 1158-11

Edgar Cayce recommended massage in thousands of readings for the treatment and prevention of a variety of ills, and as an aid in gaining a higher level of well-being. Cayce's health readings are still being investigated because of their proven effectiveness. They continue to grow more widely acclaimed by lay persons and health care providers, including medical doctors who use their recommendations.

Francis Sporer has taught at the Cayce/Reilly School of Massotherapy, at the A.R.E., Virginia Beach, Virginia, for over 13 years. He maintains that massage is more than a discretionary luxury and should be viewed as a near-necessity for wellness.

In 1982, Sporer studied with Dr. Harold Reilly, the famous physiotherapist that Cayce recommended by name in readings. He has avidly investigated and applied Cayce's readings since 1967. Sporer's classes are taught in the USA, Europe and the Orient. He teaches Cayce's holistic health concepts, remedies and the unique massage methods of the Cayce/Reilly Technique.

Sporer's most recent video, *The Cayce-Reilly Massage Technique...and Beyond,* was released in 2001. The essential Cayce/Reilly Techniques for beginners and professionals are demonstrated in the video. There is also new material from Cayce's readings and Reilly's techniques, along with Sporer's original methodology.

....

The massage aids the ganglia to receive impulse from nerve forces...

EDGAR CAYCE
Reading 2458-4

....

From the Cayce readings perspective,
the greatest values of the massage are
its benefits to the circulatory and nervous
systems, both directly and reflexively.

Eric Mein, MD
From: *KEYS TO HEALTH*

....

MASSAGE: An Interview With Francis B. Sporer, MA, AMTA, NCTMB, CMT-VA

BETTE: In Edgar Cayce's readings he referred to massage as a "rub". Is that how you would describe it, Francis?

FRANCIS: A "rub" is far too modest a term, though it was once common parlance. Massage is actually very sophisticated soft tissue manipulation for relaxation and therapeutic purposes.

BETTE: I understand that at one time people were reluctant to even speak about massage, much less get one. Why?

FRANCIS: In the past, there were many stigmas attached to massage. The popular misconceptions were that massage was a luxury for only the rich, or massage was something you only did once a year on vacation. And many people equated massage with "adult entertainment", a polite euphemism for sexual contact. These are, of course, all erroneous ideas.

BETTE: Why has the attitude toward massage changed?

FRANCIS: People's consciousness has shifted in terms of realizing the health benefits of massage, their willingness to be worked on and their interest in going into the industry as practicing professionals. Massage is the fastest growing health care profession in the United States.

BETTE: The National Institute of Mental Health recently announced that after years of scientific research, there is conclusive proof that stress and depression in females sends emergency hormones flowing into the bloodstream. This contributes to brittle bones, infections and even cancer. How does massage treat stress?

FRANCIS: Studies being conducted in Florida by Candace Pert, have shown that the soothing, rhythmic massage movements almost mesmerize the body/mind while balancing and coordinating the physical body with the mind and spirit. This results in a person being able to get back in touch with the deepest core of his/her true nature. Massage has a sedative affect that equals several hours of restful sleep and an "exercise affect" that equals a walk of several miles.

BETTE: Stanford University Medical School recently reported that since 1940 the stress level for men and women has increased by 30 times.

FRANCIS: I know of that study and statistic. The natural "fight or flight" reflex to escape great anxiety is triggered daily in high stress lifestyles keeping hormones at continual hyper-readiness. This is more appropriate for survival when facing constant mortal peril, because adrenaline, which is produced as a natural reaction to apprehension, aids in choosing whether to "fight or flee" from whatever threatens our security.

BETTE: So for people in modern society, "fight or flight" is an unhealthy option.

FRANCIS: The consequences of "fight or flight" are high stress and failing of the immune system. Massage offers an answer to reducing stress. It coordinates the voluntary, or central nervous system, which administers activities we choose to engage in. And it balances the involuntary nervous system which governs the "fight or flight" reaction to danger.

BETTE: What does massage do for the endocrine system?

FRANCIS: It stimulates and balances the endocrine system. From Cayce's viewpoint, massage is the physical connection to the chakras or auric body. The endocrine glands act as transducers, transforming one form of energy to another - in this case spiritual energy into physical energy.

BETTE: How does massage affect other systems of the body?

FRANCIS: Massage improves the functioning of the skeletal, digestive, muscular, nervous and respiratory systems of the body. It also stimulates blood vessels, which improves circulation, relieving general and specific congestion. Massage reduces the load of lactic acid and other metabolic waste by-products in tissues and muscles, eliminating or decreasing aches and pains produced through strenuous workouts or muscular activity. It also goes a long way to cleanse the body of pollutants, such as medication, heavy metals and other chemical residues.

BETTE: Are there other health benefits that massage offers?

FRANCIS: Massage stimulates lymph, which reduces edema, or swelling due to fluid retention. It improves the elasticity of the skin and stretches connective tissue to keep the body flexible. In healthy people massage enables excretion of fluids through the kidneys, facilitating the elimination of excess nitrogen, inorganic phosphorus and salt. A good abdominal massage can also facilitate more thorough elimination of fecal matter. Massage increases the manufacture of red blood cells, which is especially useful in cases of anemia. It also helps maintain muscle tone, preventing or delaying muscular atrophy which commonly occurs when lying in bed after recuperating from surgery, injury, or illness.

BETTE: Can massage compensate for lack of exercise?

FRANCIS: In part. And it can partially compensate for lack of muscular movement, in injured or ill people who are forced to remain inactive, by manually returning venous blood to the heart so strain on the vital organs is eased.

BETTE: What other conditions can massage relieve?

FRANCIS: Massage can abate restlessness, tension, insomnia and fatigue. It improves body alignment through manipulation of joints and the stretching of soft tissue. It can ease soreness and stiffness in painful muscles, joints and aching feet, and it can also increase the flexibility and range of motion in joints. Cayce said relaxing and resting the entire body, to nourish a sense of well-being, is vital for good health. Massage does all of that and more.

BETTE: I understand there are special sports massage techniques that can help improve an athlete's performance.

FRANCIS: I have used sports massage on professional performers, musicians and athletes such as Rudolf Nureyev and John McEnroe, before or between events to stimulate the body for peak performance, and prevent pulled muscle injuries, cramps and "charleyhorses". Massage dramatically increases performance, speed and ease of movement.

BETTE: Can massage reduce scar tissue?

FRANCIS: A special "cross fiber" massage technique broadens and thins scar tissue caused by torn muscle injury. This eliminates pain and restricted movement, as well as preventing further formation of adhesions and scars.

BETTE: How long do the benefits of a massage last?

FRANCIS: One can often feel its effects for at least two days, with residual calm lasting up to a week. Certain physiological benefits can sometimes be permanent. I like to think that a good therapist reembodies a client limb-by-limb. The immediate physical sensation one feels indicates the rejuvenating and refreshing qualities.

BETTE: After a massage, when toxins are eliminated as a result of increased circulation, are there side effects?

FRANCIS: A few people may feel sluggish the next day. They get what is called a "massage hangover", especially after a first massage when the typical system is loaded with toxins that are stirred up. Some people experience an additional bowel movement or two, or more frequent urination for a short time. But there is nothing wrong with any of this, in fact, it is good because it indicates that you are starting to clean up your body. Once the toxins are eliminated, people feel wonderfully revitalized.

BETTE: Would you say that massage is holistic in nature?

FRANCIS: According to Cayce, holistic health is the treatment of all four aspects of who we are as beings, physically, mentally, emotionally and spiritually. So, yes, massage addresses all of these levels of being and can be classified as holistic in nature.

BETTE: But massage cannot take the place of good diet, exercise or a meditation program for attunement to God.

FRANCIS: You are correct. Each person is responsible for the care of their body, mind, emotions and spirit. Cayce suggests that a person's health never remains status quo - it is either getting better or worse. Unless you are continually improving your whole self through diet, exercise, massage, medicine, meditation and study groups, or participation in some kind of spiritual path that contributes to your spiritual growth, you cannot expect continued healthy growth.

BETTE: So you are saying that to be healthy every aspect of us must vibrate at an equal, optimum level?

FRANCIS: Right again. Since everything in the universe is vibrational energy, you cannot change for the better by leaving any part of yourself behind at a lower vibration. For example, it is impossible to be completely healthy if you eat junk food, even if you meditate daily. Edgar Cayce's son, Hugh Lynn Cayce, warned people to get spinal adjustments from an Osteopath, work with their diet, exercise, learn to relax and uplift the different parts of their body, mind, emotions and spirit before getting involved in a serious program of spiritual growth, including meditation. This is because your total being plays a role in your vibrational self and activates the energies of the endocrine and chakra systems, especially the so-called kundalini or "serpent" force, which can actually cause harm if you are not emphatically working toward a balance of all that you are.

BETTE: The promise in the Cayce readings is that we can rejuvenate ourselves and live to be whatever age we wish. How can we accomplish that?

FRANCIS: One of the main clues that Cayce gave us was in his reading that said: ***"There should be a warning to all bodies...for would the assimilations and the eliminations be kept nearer normal in the human family, the days might be extended to whatever period as was desired; for the system is builded by the assimilations of that it takes within, and is able to bring resuscitation so long as the eliminations do not hinder."*** (3312-1)

BETTE: Please clarify that.

FRANCIS: Assimilation refers to the body's ability to absorb the nutrients from the food we give it to work with. Most people don't realize there is such a thing. They use the word "digestion" as a catch-all term for a very complex process. In order for the body to properly utilize the food we eat, we need to recognize that it includes chewing foods thoroughly, followed by the body's proper breakdown of food into constituent nutrients so that assimilation in the small intestine and internal organs can take place. Food values, such as minerals and vitamins, are stored and/or put to work to replenish the body. Elimination refers to the process of ridding the body of toxins leftover from food, emotions, attitudes or from daily activities. The process occurs through sweating through the skin, properly deep breathing through the lungs, drinking lots of water to clean out the kidneys and daily bowel movements to clear the colon. Nature's required housecleaning of the body's systems eliminates poisons and congestion that lead to illness. Massage and hydrotherapy are important tools in the preventative and curative processes of the body.

BETTE: How often did Cayce mention massage in his readings?

FRANCIS: Cayce did 14,246 readings. 64%, or 9000 of these readings dealt with health. And 75% of the 9000 health readings recommended massage in one form or another.

BETTE: How does the Cayce view of massage compare to conventional massage?

FRANCIS: For one thing, Cayce recommended 3 types of massage. The first is Swedish massage. Dr. Reilly's method is a unique form of Swedish not taught any place else. It incorporates many unique movements and concepts, some of which come directly from the Cayce readings, although most are from his own wisdom or people he considered authorities in physical therapies.

BETTE: What does Swedish massage accomplish?

FRANCIS: It reduces lactic acid build up, relieves muscle spasm and tension, stimulates circulation, aids in the elimination of metabolic wastes and congestion, and relaxes and frees movement.

BETTE: What is the second type of massage that Cayce recommended?

FRANCIS: Osteopathic Massage. It is different from osteopathic adjustment. Dr. Andrew Taylor Still, founder of Osteopathy, discovered that by touching the body in certain ways it redistributed or replenished the energies of the nervous system. Osteopathic Massage includes a form of magnetic healing which Mr. Cayce's readings also endorsed. I have found that Osteopathic Massage is tremendously useful for removing tension by doing certain forms of stretching, even while doing a regular massage. This loosens the body and gets the nervous system and blood flow functioning more efficiently. Certain forms of Chinese bodywork, such as Qi Gong Massage, are very osteopathic in nature. In fact, they have borrowed some of Dr. Still's techniques and incorporated them into Qi Gong.

BETTE: What is the third type of massage?

FRANCIS: Neuropathic Massage. But we know very little about it because all Cayce said in his readings was to go to a Neuropathic Massage specialist. He never explained what the specialist would do beyond working on the nervous system and the nervous pathways. The Meridian Institute's team of scientists, researchers and medical doctors, affiliated with the A.R.E., are trying to rediscover some of the specifics about Neuropathic Massage.

BETTE: Do you utilize what little is known of Neuropathic Massage?

FRANCIS: I utilize what I have come to be quite sure of concerning Neuropathic Massage. For instance, strokes downward from the head and outward from the midline of the body are sedating and vice versa.

BETTE: So you incorporate your own massage methods with Cayce recommended massage?

FRANCIS: Yes. The back routine I developed emphasizes certain patterns, that I insist on from students, to aid in the purpose we are trying to accomplish. I also teach specific therapeutic nervous system and muscular movements. They are focused on the 4 plexuses that Cayce spoke of, which lay on the spine: the brachial, solar, lumbar and sacral plexuses. We know that specific movements can retrain any nervous pathway that has become disoriented.

BETTE: Can you give an example?

FRANCIS: I once worked with a Viet Nam war veteran suffering from Post-Traumatic Shock Syndrome. He was a fairly extreme case of how the nervous system gets out of whack under conditions that shock the sensibility of the mind and emotions. Certain neuropathic stroking patterns given to him in a psychic health reading were administered. With only six or seven treatments he improved impressively.

BETTE: What kind of oils did Cayce suggest for massage?

FRANCIS: There are many, used singularly or mixed together, for various purposes. One combination that he said was excellent for the skin is a mixture of 6 ounces of peanut oil and 2 ounces of olive oil, 1 tablespoon of lanolin, and 2 ounces of rosewater.

BETTE: Is that the mixture you use for massage?

FRANCIS: Sometimes, depending upon the need of the client. I use a number of different formulas. As a general rule, I usually work with half peanut oil and half olive oil that I mix in a squeeze bottle. Following Cayce's recommendation, I sometimes use olive oil or peanut oil for specific reasons.

BETTE: Didn't Cayce say that peanut oil relieves arthritis?

FRANCIS: Yes, as well as many other conditions; and it works! He especially saw it as an aid to the joints. It also helps to recondition the way the liver and kidneys interact with each other, so they can function in a healthy manner. Cayce even recommended practically "bathing" in peanut oil or olive oil about twice a week. He referred to olive oil as one of the most effective agents for stimulating and rebuilding muscle and mucous membrane and the nervous system. Cayce called it a "food" for the soft tissue. So, massage is yet another form of assimilation. It helps the body absorb what it needs from the particular properties in whatever is applied to it. Only recently, medical science finally came to accept what the readings affirmed years before, that the body readily absorbs substances through the skin. The readings also assert that massage is an important way to expedite this process.

BETTE: How do you apply the oils you use?

FRANCIS: Initially it is always done lightly, to initiate touch to warm up the body part, and to coat the skin surface. Long strokes called "effleurage" are done toward the heart, which protects the veins from damage. Thereafter I perform the techniques I decide on for that limb or body part. When I massage the back, standing at the head, I apply oil straight down the spine about 6 or 7 times, returning up the sides of the body in a fairly slow movement to start setting up the "Relaxation Response" in the whole central nervous system. The acceptance of this Neuropathic Massage technique has been established by the research of Herbert Benson, MD, Harvard University School of Medicine. Dr. Benson did research in the 60s, revealing that meditation slows the pulse, lowers blood pressure, slows breathing and relaxes muscles. Since massage does all of these things too, it accomplishes the same "Relaxation Response".

BETTE: Do you have any special remedies that you use for strained or sprained muscles?

FRANCIS: The best thing for muscle strains is Cayce's remedy of a "pack" made with sea salt and apple cider vinegar. It is incredibly effective for any strain or sprain. I have seen this pack cure a serious knee sprain for the 80-year-old father of one of my best friends. Cayce's old stand-by, castor oil packs, are very good for relieving muscle strains and sprains too. Castor oil speeds up the lymphatic cleansing process, carries away injured cells and increases "T" cells which accelerates the healing process. Once, I completely cleared up my acute ankle sprain overnight by sleeping with a castor oil-soaked wool sock on it. I also use the formula with kerosene in it that the readings recommended. It can be purchased commercially, in a premixed formula under the brand name:

Muscle Treat (tm)
From: the Heritage Store, Virginia Beach, VA
(www.heritagestore.com)
Phone: 1-800-862-2923)

or under the brand name:

Myo-Relief tm
From: Barr Products
(www.baar.com)
Phone: 1-800-269-2502

BETTE: I've heard that olive oil taken internally is good for the stomach.

FRANCIS: Absolutely. Take only 1/4 to 1/2 teaspoon of olive oil on an empty stomach, one to five times a day. "Chew" it a bit at first, as the readings say. This eliminates gas formation and prevents an upset stomach. Cayce emphasized that only a small amount be taken, because small amounts are what the body can absorb at one time. There's a clue here about assimilation. From a Cayce viewpoint, more is not better for the body because assimilation can only take place at a certain rate. Putting too much of even good things into the body will make it impossible for the body to utilize. For example, one-fourth of a glass of freshly squeezed orange juice, slowly sipped over a 10-minute period, is better for assimilation than gulping down a quart of it, which will compromise assimilation.

BETTE: Is there a particular brand of oil that you recommend?

FRANCIS: Cayce said "pure" olive oil which means the first pressing ("virgin" or "extra-virgin" designations). Purity also means that it does not have herbicides or pesticides in it. My understanding of supermarket peanut oils is that they often contain rancid peanuts that are squeezed and chemically cleaned up a bit. Buy quality organic, cold-pressed oils at a health food store. Cold pressing preserves the enzymes and the integrity of the oil, as opposed to fast grinding processes that generate heat which destroys these properties.

BETTE: Cayce's readings recommend different massage protocols for various people. What were those protocols?

FRANCIS: The techniques given in readings were often in a limited form that would help an individual with particular problems. However, Cayce also recommended general, full-body massage, usually Swedish style, as being beneficial for nearly everyone. One reading recipient asked about specific techniques that he should seek from a massage therapist. Cayce's answer was to get the massage and leave the method and techniques to the massage therapist. The readings gave very specific procedures for work alongside the spine in order to bring about coordination between the central and autonomic nervous systems.

BETTE: What happens to the body when there is discoordination between the central and autonomic nervous systems?

FRANCIS: Discoordination between the autonomic, or involuntary nervous system, with its sympathetic and parasympathetic branches, and the central, or voluntary nervous system, is the leading cause of dis-ease according to the readings. Dis-ease leads to disease. Discoordination means that the two systems are not communicating nor interacting with each other. The old adage about a house divided against itself is apropos here.

BETTE: How can this be prevented?

FRANCIS: Well, as the saying goes, "Life Happens." Perhaps we can't prevent it, but we can correct it. Cayce described four patterns that could bring about the desired coordination, however, two were given for extremely limited application. And one is too complicated and time-consuming for most people to learn. The fourth, which was recommended more frequently than the others, is helpful to everyone and is the one Dr. Reilly emphasized. It involves using finger or thumb tips just on either side of the spine, starting at the neck, and moving in an upward and outward circular, spiraling manner as you progress downward. I think of tracing little hearts on each side of the spine as I move downward.

BETTE: What would the ideal massage protocol be?

FRANCIS: I'm not sure there is only one ideal protocol. But to have a massage in the morning, thoroughly working the whole spine, would be my idea of a perfect world. Cayce said: ***"...this would stimulate, enliven and coordinate the whole nervous system, and the four nerve plexuses located in the torso - the brachial, solar, lumbar and sacral - using olive oil. Or, equal parts of tincture of myrrh and olive oil which strengthens the body overall."*** (5421-6) Using this combination, the oil must be heated first, then the myrrh is added to it.

BETTE: Can you give some of Cayce's theory about these nerve plexuses?

FRANCIS: Cayce talked about the nerve center locations as areas in the nervous system, at certain places on the spine, that contain a major aggregation of brain-like nerves. They emerge from that spinal region branching into, and governing, certain portions of the body. Directly connecting to the endocrine gland and the chakra they interface with, they each form a bridge from the infinite to the finite parts of ourselves, acting as the transducers of energy we mentioned earlier.

BETTE: So the nerve plexuses' function is to regulate the body through the power of hormonal secretions?

FRANCIS: Yes. And they reflect our karma, or memory patterns stored in the DNA, and send us imagery, especially in non-ordinary states, like when we are dreaming or under the influence of drugs, during meditation or in reveries. That is why Cayce recommended that a physician who came for a reading, study the *Book of Revelation.* The psychological, spiritual, archetypal, emotional and physiological aspects of self were all interacting in a way that enabled John, the Beloved Disciple, to "see" symbolically what was going on at that moment in his consciousness and in his body. The imagery was all playing on his inner movie screen.

BETTE: What did Cayce mean when he referred to these nerve centers as "vegetative brains"?

FRANCIS: "Vegetative brains" refers to the automatic functioning of these nerve centers, unless directed from higher sources to do otherwise. Each plexus/

gland/chakra has a territory to govern, and an agenda of its own, regarding the well-being of its particular section of the body. Each is like a minister in a federal government with a task to supervise. They are supposed to work under the direction of the head of government which would be the pituitary, pineal and thyroid functioning as one. However, unless they are directed by these three higher spiritual centers, which taken together form a higher spiritually-purposed way of doing things, they will function piecemeal, and automatically based on their previous conditioning, memory or karma. This can, however, be way off-base. No wonder we get out of coordination and sick!

BETTE: Are there techniques to prevent this incoordination?

FRANCIS: Cayce said we must have an ideal by which we make decisions. Our ideal is based on what we have studied, what we believe, and what we have applied. Then we must choose to put our higher choices into action and make sure the "ministers" reflect that as they govern their territories. Cayce also said that if we live in harmony with our ideal we will experience good health, peace of mind and the abundance of the Creative Forces (a name Cayce used interchangeably with "God"). That is why a heavy smoker, for example, could live to a ripe old age and never suffer the ill effects others do. Of course, it's easy to justify our choices by saying we are living in harmony with our ideal. But the Higher Self is ultimately the final authority on that, not our ego or conscious selves.

BETTE: Can you give an illustration of the Higher Self as the final authority?

FRANCIS: The brachial plexus, which is located in the vicinity of T-1 to T-4 , ("T" meaning the "thoracic" portion of the spine), governs the heart, lungs, arms, hands - the whole upper torso. The "Ministry of the Brachial Plexus" involves the heart chakra and the thymus endocrine gland with its powerful and vital hormonal secretions that regulate the immune system. The minister reacts to outside stimuli with our conditioned response version of "love consciousness" - which is what the heart center is all about. Our health, especially in that region of the body, depends on what we understand to be the highest way of showing love in our lives. It causes our subjective karmic reactions to kick in, revolving around issues of affection and healing. This is our subconscious mind at work. Love encompasses not only positive feelings like altruism and unconditional acceptance, but also possessiveness, sentimentality, jealousy, "smother" love and an assortment of other negative manifestations. We can see that we have work to do when illness strikes, as illness, a form of dis-ease, can reflect our imperfect understanding of love.

BETTE: You have just given a brief description of Cayce's holistic approach to physical, mental, spiritual and emotional well-being and personal evolvement.

FRANCIS: We are "one" in our "beingness". The physical, mental, emotional and spiritual parts of which we are composed, are a reality, not merely discrete or theoretical concepts. Dreams, synchronicities, challenges, opportunities, people and events are all involved in our physiological functioning. Dream imagery, for example, can give us pictures of physical conditions. And our karma actually creates the pattern of our DNA as gestation of the fetus takes place.

BETTE: How does massage fit into this body/mind concept?

FRANCIS: Massage upon, and outward from these plexuses stimulates the nerve branches connecting the cerebrospinal, and sympathetic ganglia. It coordinates the activities among these nerve centers and helps to make them work in relationship to each other so there is a oneness or holism going on in the body. In the massage that I do, I pay particular attention to these areas cited by Cayce, to try and assure that nerve impulses are correctly activated and directed through patterns used when touching the body.

BETTE: Can you recommend message that can be done at home?

FRANCIS: If it's tender to the touch and isn't an injury, by all means, touch it. A comfortable pressure with a fingertip or pencil eraser can activate the healing mechanisms in a sore area. Acupressure is immensely powerful. Also effective for at-home massage is the Cayce head-and-neck exercise, a form of massage that most A.R.E. members know how to do. It's easy to find that method described in books such as *The Edgar Cayce Handbook for Health Through Drugless Therapy*, by Dr. Reilly. This book also includes diagrams for self massage.

BETTE: Can the spinal massage technique that you described earlier be done at home?

FRANCIS: It can easily be done, but requires two people, of course. The one receiving the massage can sit backwards on a chair with no arms, leaning forward against the back support. Put a pillow between the body and the chair for comfort. The other person giving the massage, sits facing the person's exposed back, applies some oil and draws those little hearts from top to bottom in a continuing spiral. The fingertips on the left hand draw the left half of the heart and vice versa. Beyond these techniques, I would recommend obtaining a good Cayce/Reilly technique oriented massage video and applying the demonstrated methodology. (*See recommended videos at the end of chapter*).

BETTE: I assume that home massage is not nearly as effective as a massage done by a professional therapist?

FRANCIS: Probably not, but it is better than none. And there is no reason anyone reasonably good with their hands can't learn some basic techniques that are relaxing and helpful. When Dr. Reilly devised his basic technique, he intended for it to provide continuing care for those who are ill or in need of a massage. He openly reinforced the Cayce readings which state that someone who cares about the person they are working on, can be better than an emotionally detached professional.

BETTE: Did Dr. Reilly teach laymen how to administer massage to family members?

FRANCIS: He did. In five two-hour sessions, Dr. Reilly taught family members a simple set of massage techniques so they could assist in their loved one's healing when no one else was available. These techniques are now taught at the Cayce/Reilly School of Massotherapy at the beginning of a student's training. In reading 5467-1, Cayce was asked, ***"Who should give the massage?*** His reply was, ***"One that is in attune with that (which) is being attempted."*** Almost anyone can acquire skills, but there is no substitute for the power and energy of love.

....

Contact Francis Sporer at:

Phone: 757-340-1996
Email: Tingo123@aol.com

RECOMMENDED READING

All books and tapes are available
from the A.R.E. Press
1-800-ARE-0050

....

EDGAR CAYCE'S HANDBOOK FOR HEALTH
THROUGH DRUGLESS THERAPY
Harold J. Reilly, MD
A.R.E. Press, 1989

EDGAR CAYCE'S MASSAGE,
HYDROTHERAPY AND HEALING OILS:
Health Through Coordination and
Purification of Key Body Systems
Joseph Duggan, Ms. T. and Sandra Duggan, RN
Inner Vision Publishing, 1995

VIDEOTAPES:

MASSAGE FOR BEGINNERS:
A Cayce/Reilly Video Workshop
Vicki Battaglia
A.R.E. Press, 1991

THE CAYCE/REILLY TECHNIQUE
...AND BEYOND:
For Beginners and Professionals
Francis Sporer, 2001
Also available via:
Email: Tingo123@aol.com
Phone: 1-757-340-1996

13

PAST LIFE REGRESSION
A Workshop With Sandee Mac, Past Life Regression Therapist

....

...Each soul or entity will and does return... as does nature in its manifestations about man...Life...is continuous.

EDGAR CAYCE
Reading 938-1

Sandee Mac is a well known regression therapist, spiritual counselor and teacher. After graduating from Sam Houston College in the late 60s, she worked as a psychiatric social worker in a 200 bed mental hospital. Mac was disillusioned with the mental health system in this country because she rarely saw patients get better. She left her job, moved to Europe, and during her 4 years abroad, Mac began to expand on her lifelong studies in spiritual teachings and metaphysical principles. Upon her return to the States, she read Dick Sutphen's, *You Were Born Again To Be Together* and *Past Lives, Future Lives*, classics in the field of reincarnation and past life regression. Sutphen had developed effective hypnotherapy methodology to facilitate people into past life regression. Mac became Sutphen's student because she was impressed with his idea of using regression therapeutically to access past lives that affected present life problems. She learned his regression techniques and opened her practice as a regression therapist. Mac has helped thousands of people recall past life memories as a means of comprehending themselves and deciphering their soul's purpose in this lifetime. Her techniques include integrating hypnotic trance regression with her extensive knowledge of spiritual teachings and metaphysical principles. Mac was featured in Rosemary Guiley's book, *Tales of Reincarnation.*

Know, so long as we feel there is karma, it is cause and effect.
But in righteousness we may be justified before the Throne;
Thus we may pass from cause and effect, or karma, to that of grace.

EDGAR CAYCE
Reading 3177-1

....

PART ONE - INTRODUCTION
Past Life Regression Workshop
With Sandee Mac

I am at Center Point, a spiritually-based, non-profit educational center in Houston, Texas. Hypnotherapist Sandee Mac is conducting a class on past-life regression. There are 25 people in attendance. They are seated on the floor, some on pillows, others on blankets that they have brought with them. Ms. Mac begins by explaining her understanding of past life regression, group regression, reincarnation and what can be expected during a regression:

She says: "Reincarnation is the capacity for the soul, which is eternal, to take on at intervals lifetime after lifetime in another body and in another experience of being in physical form. Each incarnation provides an opportunity to attain a higher level of soul growth through lessons learned in life. According to the universal law of karma, what we reap in one lifetime is what we sow in another. But karmic debts can be forgiven if we vibrate at a level of love, forgiveness, compassion and nonjudgement. Ultimately, that is what we are all here for, until we reach more awareness of our connection with God, or experience an aspect of the Divine, like the limitation of being in physical form.

"The soul can also reincarnate on other plane levels and dimensions. It does not have to be in a physical body. However, in 25 years of regressing thousands of people, I have met fewer than a dozen clients who have not had former lifetimes on the earth plane or only a small number of karmic issues to balance. In most cases, the few who are part of this limited category are very advanced souls who came here to teach, inspire and help others. It is useful to remember that the soul chooses the dimension level and circumstances it wishes to incarnate into. And it can bring gifts, talents, capabilities, knowledge and special qualities that were earned or highly developed as a result of discipline, study, or wisdom from prior lifetimes.

"It is my understanding as a conscious entity that the earth is moving to a higher stage on its own spiral of growth. As we move through the 4th and perhaps the 5th dimension, the opportunity for souls to reincarnate back on the earth plane will be limited to those who have achieved a certain level of higher consciousness. As a result, there will no longer be the degree of abuse, violence, suffering and negativity that was and is on our earth plane. Souls who reincarnate back to this planet will be of a higher frequency or vibration. And souls that still need a low vibration experience of negativity, violence or abuse on others will reincarnate on planets other than earth where they can continue with their evolvement.

"Past life regression is a hypnosis technique or therapy that enables a person to enter an extended state of consciousness and access impressions and memories from their other lifetimes. This can also occur through spontaneous regression, an unprompted visualization of events that took place in one's other lifetimes. Sometimes experiences in the present trigger spontaneous regression. Memories from a former incarnation are often delivered through one's dreams. A visit to a particular place may provoke deja'vu, inducing strong convictions that a previous lifetime was lived in that area. Spontaneous regression may also be aroused by meeting someone you feel strongly connected to or repulsed by. Fears, phobias and health problems may also provide karmic clues to past lives that can be verified during regression.

"Several years ago I regressed a man in Nevada who had accessed the memory of his skills from another lifetime. I met him while visiting a friend who lives in Nevada. While I was there, I saw some private appointments, and he was one of them. During his hypnotic trance I found that he had known my friend in Atlantis where he had been the equivalent of a doctor of chiropractic. While in regression, I asked him to assume the personality of the person he was in Atlantis. I explained that he would still be in an altered state of consciousness, although his eyes would be open and he would be able to move around the room.

"My friend was there during the regression, and he was able to identify places in her back and specific vertebrae where there were difficulties. He made recommendations from the perspective of the physician that he had been in Atlantis. In the present lifetime, this young man had no medical training or background in healing. Yet the information he gave related accurately to what my friend had been told about her back problems by her physicians. His recommendations as the Atlantean doctor were very unique. He suggested a water exercise in which she would float on a bag made of the carcass of an animal, such as a bull that had been sewn shut so it would still float like an inner tube.

"I have seen people who have reincarnated with specific astrological propensities, a preference for the family they wish to be born into, as male in one lifetime and female or bisexual in other incarnations, past life genetic propensities, chronic and acute health problems that they have brought with them from other lifetimes, birth marks or scars from wounds received in a past life and karmic soul deficits. Often we think of karma as a negative quality. However, karma, or destiny of the soul, is neither a punishment nor a reward system. Instead, it is an opportunity to optimize the journey of the soul's growth by correcting mental, emotional, physical and spiritual patterns that do not manifest in alignment with harmony or God's Law of Love. Of course, all religions have their own strong opinion about what this means. For me, personally, I simply ask, 'Does it support the order of life, or not?'

"Karmic force enables the soul to experience various approaches of perception from one lifetime to another. For example, a number of my clients were in W.W.II, died and then reincarnated. Sometimes Germans come back as Jews and Jews reincarnate as Germans. That is always surprising and in some cases shocking to them. I have also regressed young people in their late teens or early 20s who have had previous incarnations in Viet Nam, lost their lives there and then reincarnated, bringing the same soul deficiencies with them from their former lives. I have regressed numerous young people who died of drug problems in the 60s and are now back picking up where they left off, so to speak.

"One of my most interesting clients was a young man who fought in Viet Nam in his last life. He came to a group regression that his high school teacher had arranged for him. In trance, he accessed particularly vivid and insightful memories of what he experienced in Viet Nam. During a subsequent private regression with me, he revealed his many lifetimes at war, including one in Roman times, another at the time of the Civil War and the most recent in Viet Nam. He was the kind of person that authors write books about on past life regression because he got such exquisite details of himself as a warrior, fighter and soldier. While he was in hypnosis, I asked him about his lifetime in Viet Nam. He said that he had been an American soldier and he told me his entire name and rank. I asked him to look down and read the serial number on his dogtag. As he read it, I wrote it down. He told me that he was shot and killed in Viet Nam. In his present life, his father had connections at the Pentagon, so he was able to verify the name and dogtag number he had given during his regression. They matched exactly to the Pentagon records. Shortly after his regression, he made a trip to Washington, DC where he found his name on the Viet Nam Memorial Wall. When asked what his karmic lesson was from his past lives, the information he gave in trance was that war is not the answer to conflict, and we need to find other ways to develop peace and solve planetary problems. He was certain that in his present lifetime he did not want military activity or violence of any kind because of the knowledge he acquired at war in his past incarnations.

"Past life regression is also therapeutically helpful for people struggling with substance abuse. In most cases they have had past lives as addicts, died as a result of their substance abuse and reincarnated into the present lifetime with the same chemical dependency. Going back and viewing previous lives where the same difficult chronic problems existed seems to support and accelerate the soul in clearing detrimental patterns in the present lifetime.

"I regressed a client who had a chronic history of substance abuse that he eventually conquered in this life experience. At the time of regression he looked at his multiple past lives in which he was obsessed with alcohol and drugs. In his present life he had been adopted at birth. His adoptive father was an alcoholic, so one might assume he learned his behavior from his adoptive father. He was able to access his birth records from a Dallas, Texas adoption agency only to discover that his birth parents were alcoholics too. So he was genetically predisposed to work with substance abuse in this lifetime.

"I have found that most adopted children have had past lives with their adoptive parents. In many cases they have not had any or very many incarnations with their biological parents. Often, they have had past lives where they lost, abandoned or gave up their biological children. Such was the case with this young man in a number of his past lives. Reincarnating as a person who was abandoned at birth and grew up to become an alcoholic, presented him with an opportunity to adjust his soul's knowledge by experiencing abandonment as his past life biological children did. He also had the chance to finally overcome his multi lifetimes as an alcoholic. It was very rewarding when he overcame his karmic substance abuse to become a drug and alcohol counselor. He dedicated his present life to supporting other addicts on their path to recovery and soul growth.

"My parents introduced me to Edgar Cayce's reincarnation concepts when I was about 11 years old. I remember them reading *There is a River*, and then sending the book to friends and relatives because they wanted to share Cayce's revelations. His depiction of reincarnation made sense to me, especially in light of a family trip we made to the Rio Grande Valley of Texas when I was 10 years old. It was there that I came face to face with extreme poverty. I never forgot the unbearable sight of flies clinging to the bodies of crippled, starving beggars on the streets of the Mexican border towns. My family and school teachers taught me that everyone was created equal, but I could see that was not so. I was stunned and disappointment about how unjust and inequitable life seemed to be. But Cayce's explanation of reincarnation offered a deeper understanding of reality. What appeared to be a harsh fate for some people was explicable in terms of karma and soul evolution. I can now view human suffering with great compassion, and realize that despite one's karmic debts, we still need to take action and work to improve the circumstances of people in need.

"Cayce's readings and my mentor Dick Sutphen have taught me to look for karmic motivation behind a client's inclination to be a particular way. I have been trained to ask: how do a client's present circumstances tie in with universal karmic law and their conduct in past lives? How is the soul trying to achieve companionship with God? How can I support my client in understanding the opportunities that are presented in this lifetime, in order to evolve to a higher, loving, compassionate nonjudgmental awareness? And how can I help my client to see that their current circumstances were created by them, not so they can feel like a victim of life, but for the opportunity of soul growth?

"As a Virgo, my propensity in this lifetime is to help people. It is a disposition related to two of my past lives. I discovered that in some of my previous incarnations I had issues of abuse and use of power. Therefore, a large part of my greater soul objective in this lifetime is to utilize my capabilities to support people in finding direction on a path that clears out and resolves old issues so they can experience attunement with God. Another part of my purpose is to assist people in comprehending and getting ready for earth changes that are happening and also drawing near. One of my past lives was in Atlantis when I was involved with preparing people to flee before the cataclysmic changes occurred. However, I did not make provisions for my own escape. This accounts for my sense of urgency in this lifetime about planning for adverse earth changes. During W.W.II, in a lifetime when I was part of the French Resistance, I guided people in escaping Nazi Germany. In that lifetime, I died a year before the war was over and reincarnated in my present lifetime a year after the war ended in 1946. I have always felt a very strong connection with Europe and W.W.II. As a young girl I read *Anne Frank: Diary of a Young Girl,* which made a significant impression on me. Last year, I made a trip to Germany where I worked on the release of old judgments, fears, suspicions and doubts that I had during WW II.

"I have found that certain patterns perpetuate themselves. For example, almost all abused, molested or incested people in this life were perpetrators in a past life. Regression permits a client to look at their past lives as victims or perpetrators, or in most cases, both. This is a liberating process from the victim role. It blows the lid off a lot of therapeutic practices, because in trance the client realizes that current predicaments are something they chose for themselves to improve the soul. In almost every case of victim /perpetrator abuse, I have noted that whatever abuse committed on a person in the present lifetime is minimal, or to a much smaller degree, compared to what they did to others in past lifetimes. For example, a man who was a ruthless abuser in past lifetimes, may reincarnate as a woman who is molested by her father in this lifetime, but not necessarily in an extremely violent way, although I have run into that as well.

"I have also treated many families who while in trance learned that they exchanged roles in various lifetimes, reincarnating back with their own families after their death. For example, I regressed a client who was once a grandparent, then died and reincarnated back into her own family as her own grandchild. I also regressed a father in one lifetime who incarnated as a sister with reincarnated family members from a former lifetime. Often, spouses, good friends, lovers or enemies from past lives incarnate as people who are still connected in a new lifetime. I have even had clients who reincarnated more than once with their pets in order to learn and grow from them.

"Lost souls and discarnate entities, is another realm that I have worked with extensively. In some cases I have regressed an entity so it can understand how it got stuck between lifetimes, especially if it is in an area that is affecting a particular physical location or another person's energy field. Often an entity doesn't know their physical body has died. I have learned a lot from discarnate entities and developed some very simple and effective techniques so they can find their way from this dimension to the next and move on to higher levels of awareness.

"My sessions with clients are taped and usually last about 1-1/2 to 2 hours, at which time we can cover up to 10 or more lifetimes. I usually try to orient the session towards discerning the past life cause of problems in this lifetime. Some people come to me because they are just curious. In this case, I will ask broad generic questions and try to get in touch with areas of personal interest that affect the present life. I may ask questions about time periods in history of particular interest to the client, or about geographic areas that they feel familiar with or have been drawn to even if they have never visited there in the present. I try to orient individual regressions around a client's strongest interests, talents and skills because these attributes are often clues to past lives. If they are coming in with a highly charged topic, I will begin by reviewing one or two of their past lifetimes where no huge emotional encumbrance exists. Then I am able to get a clear idea of how they receive information. When a chronic intense emotional plight is present, I will often have a lot of interaction with the client. While they are in trance, I guide them through forgiveness, release, review of the situation and letting go of the matter. Sometimes I take them back to the time before they were born, in that traumatic lifetime, so they can see what their soul's lesson plan was when they set themselves up to come into their present circumstances. Then they can consider if they have accomplished what they came for in a way that can allow them to let go of the negative pattern, or to ascertain what else needs to be done in order to free themselves of the predicament with love, forgiveness, compassion and nonjudgment.

"I am not a psychic, medium or channel, so I cannot see or perceive what memories and impressions a person is accessing during a regression. Therefore, I must depend on what the client tells me, as well as interpret their non-verbal signals about what they are actually perceiving in trance. As a therapist I do not have to tell the client my impressions about what happened, although I often relate details they may not have seen.

"A group regression is conducted using the same hypnosis techniques as in a regression with one person. The group can be as small as 2 or as large as 1000 people. Usually group regressions are oriented toward a general subject rather then specific questions to allow a greater number of people to be able to access impressions. People in group regressions do not ordinarily speak out loud and talk back and forth with the therapist about memories of their past lives like a person would do in an individualized session. There are unique exceptions with small private prearranged group regressions consisting of people who have shared lifetimes together. In this situation they all hear what everyone else is accessing. I may speak with them individually if they all regress to the same life time simultaneously. I did this in a group regression with people in Houston who worked together at a foundation for polio research and felt very strongly connected. While in trance they learned that in the Middle Ages they had a past life together as monks working in a monastery creating illuminated manuscripts. They were very close in that lifetime too."

PART TWO
Group Hypnosis

During the second part of the workshop, Mac addresses the concerns of the audience about hypnosis. She says:

"For those who have never done hypnosis before, be mindful that you are not going to pass into unconsciousness, become comatatose, be asleep, turn into a zombie or go back to the 1800s and be lost in time forever. If you feel anxiety before a regression, it may be because you fear the unknown, or because your subconscious senses that you are going to come up with profound information. In some cases anxiety before a regression is due to a discarnate entity around you. But usually being regressed is a comfortable experience akin to the alpha state, the condition you are in when you first wake up in the morning or when you are drowsy in the evening but not completely asleep or awake. The alpha state is the place where people go in dreams, meditation and prayer. During regression the body will be very relaxed, and the mind will be aware, alert and focused on the life experience that we are working with. I use a standard hypnotic progressive relaxation technique, relaxing the body while I count backwards from 7 to 1. I bring in some visualized protection light that will shelter you and I offer a self-release mechanism. It is very important to understand that you are perfectly safe, in control and can withdraw yourself from the altered state at any time that you choose to. The self-release mechanism gives most people a sense of security so they are able to go into a deeper trance and access memories more effectively.

"I usually use a classic hypnosis verbal induction of progressive relaxation, which means that I inform you that you are going to feel relaxed. Then I will have you imagine a pleasant situation where you are walking, riding, floating or drifting downward. I will count backwards a couple of times from 7 to 1, and then you will be under. A part of you may question it and say that you don't feel like you are in trance; but you are. I will have you imagine a tunnel. If you don't like dark places, it is best to choose a light tunnel. I will guide you through that tunnel as I count backwards from 5 to 1 and explain that when you come out of the tunnel you will be in another lifetime in another place. And you will begin to get images of yourself in that lifetime as another person. In the beginning, if you are not getting clear information, I will tell you to make it up for a minute; then it will start getting turned on and the actual impressions of your past lives will come in. We'll go through the various stages of your past life and I will ask you who you were, where you were, what was going on, what was important, who were the significant people in your life and what were the important events that occurred. I will lead you to the last day of that lifetime and see how you died.

"One of the valuable things about doing this is that you will discover that the process of death can be a very peaceful, pleasant transition. Then you will be in what we can loosely call your "Higher Self" or "Spirit Self". You will be able to observe that lifetime, be aware of why it was important, what you were working on and what was happening then. You will evaluate yourself from an observer perspective. I may have you communicate with the person you were in that lifetime to find out what happened then that relates to the present time. It could be a talent, ability, skill or something that you developed in that incarnation that is being used or developed presently. Also it might be that someone you knew from that past life is a key person in the present lifetime. Or it could be about a mistake that you made then, and now have an opportunity to rectify in this life.

"I will tell you to step back, clear it out and change past memories. That is the way I differ from many regressionists, because I do not allow my clients to access information without using it to transcend time and space and make changes in their past lives. From my years of Shamanic studies, I know that we can view and interact with time not just as linear, but also as circular, and we can step into this place to make changes. I believe that by rescripting your past lives, you can alter your current and future lifetimes. I will then guide you through forgiveness, release of the predicaments from the past, and direct you to allow that new energy to move into the present time. You may feel like you are living that past life. Some people even visualize their memories as though it was a movie, slides, a dream or floating images. Hearing, smelling or tasting information are other ways my clients have connected to their past lives. Some people will only see black because they cannot connect to visual images of their past lives. They will need to rely on their feelings and intuitions during regression and trust them.

"You can go forward and backward in time. And you can also detach, dissociate and float up above your recollections. Or you can bring yourself completely out of trance at any time that you want to, especially if you are experiencing a highly emotional situation which you find hard to handle. Nobody has to relive trauma during hypnosis. Hopefully you will remember everything. Sometimes, after a regression, people connect with memories in their dreams, meditations or intuitive awareness.

"If you wish to, you may lie down during the regression. But if you are extremely tired, you might want to sit up and lean against the wall because your body may get the message that you want to sleep. In case you fall asleep and snore loudly, it will be hard for other people in the group to make sense of that noise. So if somebody next to you is snoring, please nudge them a bit, but don't scare them out of that lifetime. And if somebody is nudging you, it probably is because you are the one snoring.

"I am going to do a group regression now, and will begin by turning the lights out and playing soft, meditation music. Please allow yourself to close your eyes, and do some deep breathing, slow and easy. Notice as you breathe deeply that you are beginning to relax completely. Slow down your thoughts. You can keep your full attention on the sound of my voice. If outside thoughts or noise comes in, brush it aside and return your concentration to the sound of my voice, breathing deeply, relaxing completely and going into a deeper state.

"We will start now. You can feel your body relaxing, one part at a time, first into your toes, then moving up your legs to your knees, relaxation into all the muscles, traveling to your thighs, your hips, taking you deeper and deeper. And you are just as deep and just as comfortable as you need to be. Your full attention is on the sound of my voice as the relaxing feeling comes into your fingers of both your hands, at the same time moving up into your forearms and your upper arms and shoulder muscles. The base of your spine feels very comfortable as the relaxation moves up to the back of your neck into your scalp. Feel your scalp relaxing and feel the tranquillity reaching your facial muscles and relaxing your jaws, your throat, your teeth. Your entire body is completely calm all over. All tension is gone from your body and mind. You feel balanced, centered and very focused.

"Begin to visualize a large, warm, white light coming down from above, entering your head and surrounding all of you. The light goes into your body and emerges from your heart center as a beautiful golden white light totally surrounding and filling your entire body, mind and soul. You are completely protected. Know that the light extends out and touches all the others in the room with you, enclosing all of us in a bubble of brilliant Divine white light. The light is grounded and connected deep into the earth and aligned through each and every order of the angels, all the way to the throne of God, the one infinite creator of love and light, protected through the order of Michael. Only your own guides, angels and master teachers, who are there for your highest and best spiritual good, will be allowed to influence you in any way. But you are now, and always are, and will always be very protected by them.

"Imagine that you are in a pleasant situation going downward, walking, or riding, or floating, or drifting down, down, down, going deeper and deeper. I will count backwards from 7 to 1, and by the time I get to number 1 you will be in a profoundly deep, very peaceful, relaxed, altered state. Imagine going down. Number 7, deeper, deeper, deeper, down, down, down. Number 6, deeper, deeper, deeper, down, down, down. Number 5, deeper, deeper, deeper, down, down, down. Number 4, deeper, deeper, deeper, down, down, down. Number 3, deeper, deeper, deeper, down, down, down. Number 2, deeper, deeper, deeper, down, down, down. Number one. Relax. Your body and mind are relaxed. Let yourself go even deeper, much, much, deeper. Think of the word "peace".

Create a situation in your mind that is totally peaceful to you and let your body, mind and spirit become part of that scene. Feel a quietness of spirit and mind. You are at peace, deeply at peace, with yourself and everyone else and the world. Carry this feeling for the rest of the evening and the days that follow. Right now you are very deep. And you are going much deeper once again, seeing and feeling yourself going down, as I count backwards from 7 to 1. By the time I get to 1 you will be in the deepest possible hypnotic state, deeper than you have ever been before. So imagine going down. Number 7, deeper, deeper, deeper, down, down, down. Number 6, deeper, deeper, deeper; down, down, down. Number 5, deeper, deeper, deeper; down, down, down. Number 4, deeper, deeper, deeper, down, down, down. Number 3, deeper, deeper, deeper, down, down, down. Number 2, deeper, deeper, deeper, down, down, down. Number 1. Your mind and body are completely relaxed. You are totally open to positive suggestion. I am going to give you two suggestions. The first suggestion is that each and every time you are hypnotized you consciously desire to be hypnotized. You will go down deeper and faster than the time before. And each time you will go far deeper and far faster than the time before. The second suggestion is that if at any time you are uncomfortable in any way, you have the power and ability to remove yourself from hypnosis.

"You can move yourself forward or backward in time. You can detach and see from the observer perspective, or if you choose, you can completely remove yourself from the altered state. You are now and for the remainder of this life in complete control to remove yourself from any kind of hypnosis or altered state you ever find yourself in. You are in control. And you are completely relaxed and at ease. Your mind is focused, calm and open to positive suggestion. In the memory banks of your subconscious is a clear recollection of everything that has ever happened to you in this life or in your past lives. Every thought, every action, every deed from any lifetime you have lived is recorded in your memory banks. We are going to work together to allow some of these memories to filter down from your subconscious into your conscious mind where you can observe them once again.

"We are now going to move backward in time to one of your previous lifetimes. I am asking your subconscious to choose a life in which you lived to be at least 30 years of age, and a lifetime that directly connects to something significant influencing your present lifetime. There may be several lifetimes that relate but your unconscious chooses the one that would be the most useful for you to re-experience at this time. Begin in your inner mind to create the impression or visualization of a tunnel. I will count backward from 5 to 1. When you come out of the tunnel you will be in another time and place with impressions of that lifetime. Begin seeing the tunnel and visualize yourself at the beginning of it. Number 5, you are stepping into the tunnel. Number 4, you begin to move backward in time. Way down at the end of the tunnel you see a light.

You are moving toward that light and on the count of 1 you will be there. At the count of 1 you will step out of the tunnel into the light. You will see yourself and receive impressions of yourself in another time and place. Number 3, you actually feel the impressions and sensation of speed as you move rapidly backwards in time. When you come out of the tunnel you will be about 15 years of age, in another time and place, in a lifetime that directly relates to your current incarnation. Number 2, you are getting very, very close. On the next count you will see, feel, or sense that you are about age 15, in a previous incarnation that is directly related and significantly important to your present lifetime. You are very close now; you are almost there. Allow it to happen. Feel it happening at the next count. Number 1, you are there now. Step out of the tunnel, step into the light. Perceive yourself. Does it feel like you are indoors or outdoors? Is it day or night? Does it feel hot, cold or just comfortable? Are you alone or with other people? Take a moment and explore your surroundings. Are you in a small or large room? Is there any furniture in that room? What kind of a place is it?

"Look down at your feet. Are you wearing shoes, boots, sandals, moccasins, or are you barefoot? Notice your hands. Do they seem rough or callused? Do you work very hard? Or are your hands soft, delicate and feminine, the hands of a woman? Consider your clothing. What does it feel like? Is it heavy, course, rough? Or is it something delicate, light weight, finely made? Study your hair. Is it long, short, pulled back? Are you wearing something on your head? What color does it feel like your hair is? Are you wearing jewelry, or ornamentation? If you have not already determined your sex, be aware of whether you are male or female?

"In that same lifetime, move forward a bit. Allow some information to come in about the house or dwelling place that you live. On the count of 3 you will be there. Number 1, you move forward in time. Number 2, trust your mind and the impressions you are accessing very, very vividly. And number 1, you are now there. Explore your house or dwelling. Is it a part of a town, village or city? Or, is it by itself in the country? Be aware of the Country or geographic area that you live in. You might see it specifically or have a sense of it. I want to know where you live. What does your home or dwelling seem to be made of? Move inside and take a look around. Notice any furnishings or belongings. Notice any kind of decoration. You may or may not see others as you look around your dwelling place. Take a moment to move to your room, your personal area, the place where you sleep. Look around. Do you see a window? If so, look outside. What do you see? Do you share your room or space with someone else, or is it your own private space? Do you have siblings? Look around that space and notice something particularly important or meaningful to you, something that you cherish. It might be an object, like an article of clothing, or some special gift that someone has given you or you have earned. Be aware of what that object is and why it has exceptional meaning to you. Where did you get it? What are your living circumstances? Let that information come in clearly. What is the most important way that you spend your time? Do you go to school? Does someone come and teach you? Do you have chores or work that you do? What is the year, or date, or century that you are in? First number of the year is? Second number of the year is? Third number of the year is? And any final numbers are? What is your name? What do they call you? First letter of your name is? Second letter of your name is? Third letter of your name is? And any following letters are?

"Stay in that same lifetime, but move forward a bit, maybe six months or a year, to another scene or situation that you have experienced that will give you more information. On the count of 3 you will be there. Number 1, stay in that same lifetime but move forward in time. Number 2, trust your mind and impressions that come in more and more vividly. And number 3, you are now there. Take a moment to explore well. Understand what is happening, who is involved and why it is significant. Who is the most important other person at that time in your life? What is your relationship to that person and why are they important?

"Let go of those impressions, and move forward again in time, maybe several months, maybe several years, to a notable event or experience. On the count of 3 you will be there. Number 1, feel yourself moving forward in time. Number 2, trust the impressions as they come in more and more vividly. Number 3, you understand everything that is of importance. Take a moment and explore your memories. You have the power and ability to ask questions. What is happening? Who is involved? Why is it important? What are you learning?

"You will now move forward in time several years to another important event. Number 1, feel yourself moving forward in time. Number 2, trust the impressions coming in. Number 3, you are now there. Does it feel like you still live in the same place that you did when you were younger? How old does it feel like you are? Are you married? Do you have a family? What is happening and who is involved? Let the information flow in.

"Number 1, moving forward again to another event, another experience. Number 2, you understand everything of importance. Number 3, you are now there. I want you to be aware of the quality of the character of the person that you are in that lifetime. Are you generous, kind, compassionate, ruthless, merciful, greedy? Do people respect you? Do they fear you? How are you considered in the community and by your own family? What is your sense of yourself as a spiritual being? Are you religious or involved with some type of religious organization? Do you have a sense of personal connection with Source? What is your work in this later time of life? What is the most important way that you spend your time?

"Letting go of those impressions. Move forward or backward in time to another key or karmic situation that you experienced. Number 1, moving around in time, still in that same lifetime. Number 2, trust yourself as the impressions come in very, very vividly. Number 3, you are now there. You have the freedom as I remain quiet to explore around and ask what is important. Understand what you need to know. Letting go of those impressions now. Move to the last day of that life without any pain or emotion. You will not have died; you will not have crossed over, but it will be the last day of that incarnation on the count of 3. Number 1, feel yourself moving back in time. Number 2, understand everything that is going on and what is important. Number 3, you are now there. It is the last day of that life. About how old does it feel like you are? Do you sense that you are alone or are there others there with you? What are the circumstances going on in your life at this time? If you have an awareness that you will soon be crossing over, are you at peace with that knowledge? Are you content that you have accomplished a lot? Go ahead and cross over into spirit. Leave your physical body behind. You will be a few moments after physical death. Number 1, you are parting from your physical body. Number 2, higher and higher. Number 3. It is a few moments after physical death. Can you see your body down below, the one you just left behind? How did your body die? Were you sick, hurt, or did something bad happen? Were you simply tired, and at peace, and ready to go? Let that come in from a very objective observer viewpoint. And now you are in Higher Self and you can look down on that life. Be aware of what you were learning and what you were working on. Why was that life important? You can also be conscious of the people you knew then, who may also be part of your present lifetime, being aware that they might not look exactly the same. But you will have a sense or awareness that it is the same person. Trust your mind. Was the person that you were then the same or different from the way you are now in temperament, character, values and personality? Focus on the person that you were then. Imagine, for just a moment, that you could literally step back in time to the man or woman you were then. In your mind, talk to the person you were. Explain that you are from the future. Thank them for that lifetime, whether it was or was not filled with misery or happiness. Whatever happened in that lifetime, it significantly contributed to your soul growth. Step back and acknowledge that.. The two of you are talking, you from the past and you from the present. You will remember the conversation when you return back to full consciousness. Take a moment now and see if there is anything that needs to be healed, released, let go of, asked forgiveness for from that lifetime. Do it right now. You can now see the person you were then, and you can release that person into the light as healed, whole, healthy and strong. If it feels appropriate, embrace the person you were then, drawing that energy of who you were then into the person you are now in your present consciousness.

"And still in the same Higher Self, look down on your present incarnation from the observer higher viewpoint. See and understand the impact of the patterns from that other lifetime as it relates to the present incarnation. Allow that understanding and wisdom to come forth. See if there are any adjustments that need to be made, something that you need to increase, decrease, change, let go of, forgive, ask forgiveness for, resolve, take action on. See yourself taking those steps, and moving along a self corrected path, to be more of service, more in love, more in balance. Ask your own God, angels, teachers, or your higher self anything else that you need to know or keep in mind. It could be about the life that you just touched in on, or about something else that is an issue at this time. Ask for clarity about what you need to know, and realize that by asking, if it is not revealed immediately, it will be in a few hours, or in a day or so.

"And now I am going to bring you back into full consciousness. You are going to awaken feeling as if you had a nice refreshing nap. Your head will be clear and you will be thinking with calm, self assurance. You will feel glad to be alive, very deeply at peace with yourself, the world, and everyone in it. You will remember everything, and you will continue to receive information inside about the things you touched in on. The information may come in dreams, meditation, intuitive awareness, of how things relate. On the count of 1, open your eyes. Number 1, you are beginning to come out. You feel the lifeblood and the circulation returning to your arms and legs. Number 2, coming out, feeling good, glad to be alive. Number 3, stretching, moving around, reorienting to present time consciousness, back to present time awareness, remembering everything with great clarity. Number 4, coming back, coming back. On the next count, you will open your eyes and be wide awake and feeling very, very good, balanced and centered. Number 5, you are wide awake. Open your eyes and feel good. Number 5, wide awake, wide awake. Open your eyes and feel good."

PART THREE
My Past Life

Each person in the class is allowed several minutes to get back into their body. Mac asks us where we have been and what happened to us during the group regression. Some people begin to laugh and others cry as they share the memories they retrieved in trance. I accessed a lifetime in which I was a well known, arrogant, impish, elegant male artist. My mother and father from that lifetime are my parents once again in my present lifetime. And I have known my children, some of my friends and business acquaintances in this lifetime from my former life as an artist. I have reincarnated with certain genetic characteristics from this past lifetime: I am short in stature, have curly hair and a weak upper respiratory system. Astrologically I am a Scorpio in this life. When I was an artist in a past incarnation, I signed my paintings, Asian style, with a small illustration of a scorpion next to my name. My love for art is a constant characteristic from that previous lifetime to this one. I studied art in my present life and earned a master's degree in it. I have worked as an illustrator of books in my present life. Another attribute from my former lifetime is my sense of humor and joy in making others laugh. In my past incarnation, as an adult I was not particularly good to women. I refused to acknowledge my illegitimate child from a romantic liaison. To balance my karma in this lifetime, I was born female. My two divorces in this lifetime were karmic in nature. I learned what it is like not to have good relationships with men. Because of these encounters, and the healing that I subsequently did within myself and with others, I was able to fulfill one of the main purposes in my present incarnation: I wrote *A Heart Full of Love*, a book is for children of divorce. The book guides readers on the art of creating peace within oneself, with family, stepfamily and extended family. *A Heart Full of Love* is helping many children of divorce and their families. It is in libraries and bookstores throughout the USA, Canada and Europe. School counselors also utilize the book to help children of divorce and their families. The "ups and downs" that I have experienced in this lifetime as a single parent have served to heighten my sensitivity to the distress encountered in bad relationships. Because I gained wisdom through my experiences, I have been able to enlighten others who are seeking peaceful solutions to common problems confronted by children of divorce and their families. By helping others, I edify my soul.

Hanging on my bedroom wall is my favorite print, a portrait that I painted in the lifetime that I was a famous artist. It is a picture of a young red-haired woman named Jo who was my mistress more than 140 years ago. The original portrait hangs in the Smithsonian Institute, Washington, DC. My name in that former incarnation was James McNeil Whistler.

Sandee Mac can be contacted at:

PO Box 990
Jewett, TX 75846
Phone: 903-626-7296
or 505-577-5775

....

RECOMMENDED READING

OLD SOULS:
The Scientific Evidence for Past Lives
Tom Shroder
Simon & Shuster, 1999

EDGAR CAYCE'S STORY OF KARMA
Mary Ann Woodward
Berkeley Publishing Group, 1994

SOUL DEVELOPMENT:
Edgar Cayce's Approach for a New World
Kevin J. Todeschi
A.R.E. Press, 2000

EXPLORE YOUR PAST LIVES
(2-Tape set)
Mark Thurston, PhD and Christoper Fazel
A.R.E. Press, 1997
1-888-ARE-0050

...each grain of thought or condition is a consequence of other conditions created by self.

EDGAR CAYCE
Reading 900-2 (19)

14

PSYCHIC
Letter From Clairvoyant Catherine Campbell To Bette S. Margolis

....

In answer to the question about how the psychic
work is accomplished through Edgar Cayce's body,
Cayce, in trance, said:

"...in this [trance] state the conscious mind is under subjugation of the subconscious mind, superconscious or soul mind;...or minds that have passed into the Beyond... What is known to one subconscious mind or soul is known to another, whether conscious of the fact or not."

EDGAR CAYCE
Reading 3744-3

....

Catherine Campbell is a psychic, healer, chakra balancer and teacher of metaphysics and esoteric subjects. She lives in Dublin Ireland where she studied psychology and holistic living at UCD (University College Dublin). Campbell offers workshops on chakra balancing, numerology, spirit guides, auras, magnetic therapy, color therapy, crystals and gems, psychic abilities, auras and meditation. "I draw people to my classes who can help each other," she says.

Campbell directs energy through her hands to correct imbalances and confirms her reading of a person's chakras with a pendulum. "I get a different feeling in my hands and body for every illness, which is something I haven't been able to teach to others," says Campbell. She utilizes Edgar Cayce's health care readings, and the work of other healers, along with her own holistic health care knowledge in her practice as a healer. Campbell is a member of the World Federation of Healers. She has turned down a film offer by the BBC about her life because she likes her privacy.

....

...Edgar Cayce stated that his information was derived from essentially two sources: 1) the subconscious mind of the individual for whom he was giving the reading; and, 2) an etheric source of information called the "askashic records," which is apparently some kind of universal database for every thought, word or deed that has ever transpired in the earth...

Kevin J. Todeschi, MA
and the Editors of the A.R.E.
From: *EDGAR CAYCE'S ESP*

There are almost as many types of psychic phenomena or psychic experience as there are individuals.

EDGAR CAYCE
Reading 1135-6

Letter From Clairvoyant Catherine Campbell To Bette S. Margolis

2001 Mar 03 - 09:09

Dear Bette,

I am writing to answer your questions about what it is like to be a psychic and healer, abilities that I was born with. My Mother told me that when I was a toddler I would tell the family things that were going to happen, and I was always right. No one in my family ever questioned my clairvoyance. Until I was twelve, I assumed that everyone had the same psychic abilities that I did. My healing gifts came later in my life and grew stronger along with my psychic abilities. I have learned from experience that the more I use my psychic and healing abilities, the more powerful they become, as my foretelling of recent natural disasters attest to. I saw and predicted the big earthquake in California, the day before it happened, in the early 90s. I always know when there is a storm approaching long before the weatherman does. Last year, I knew that Ireland, England and other countries in Europe were going to be hit by floods. And this year I can see that there will be many fires, earthquakes and volcanic eruptions throughout the world.

We all have inborn psychic abilities, although most of us are not aware of these God-given gifts. Some choose to block them out because of fear of what people might think, or non-belief in themselves. I never try to prove myself to anyone concerning my psychic and healing skills - they speak for themselves. I use my abilities to help those who seek my guidance.

As a young married woman of twenty-four with two small children, I couldn't go anywhere without picking up or tuning into other people's feelings and emotions. This made my life very uncomfortable, until I found a way to switch myself off, unless I wanted to tune in. When I conduct a psychic or healing session, I am able to listen to what a client has to say and simultaneously understand their spirit, life situation and the main problems they are having or have had. I will immediately know what the person's attributes are and how they were meant to use them. I tell clients information that is for their highest good, according to what I am seeing as a psychic and a healer. Sometimes, I do spiritual mentoring by speaking to people about being careful of their thoughts, words and actions, if I know this will help them avoid a lot of heartache and pain and ultimately assist them along their life path. Also, if I see that a past life phobia, habit or unresolved issue is responsible for obstructing a person from getting on with their purpose in this lifetime, I will tell them about this so they can work on releasing the blockage. I don't do past life readings because a person is the sum total of all their incarnations, but only the present one really matters to me. However, I can see a person's face change in front of me to a past life face. In a teaching setting, I show students how to see their past lives in terms of how it has affected their present lifetime.

Although my psychism and healings are based upon my intuition, which is always accurate, I am aware of the important part that free will plays in the outcome of a person's fate. No matter how flawless my skills are, if a client chooses a different path from the one that I foresee, their life will ultimately result in a variance of my prognostication.

Often people contact me about a personal romantic relationship they are in or would like to have. They want to know if they are perfectly matched or who a perfect mate would be. Although I can answer their questions, there is always the chance that what I "see" may be altered because of choices they make according to the law of free will. Our choices create our reality, guided by the karma, or cause and effect, that we created from past lives, the genetics of our choice (i.e. we pick the family that we wish to be born into), personality which is a matter of choosing how we wish to behave in this world, our soul's purpose, which is also preplanned before we incarnate and the life path or fate we select before we come to earth. However, all the factors of our current existence can be modified because we have free will. Karmic debts can be forgiven with good deeds, through the Grace of God. Our genes do not have to ruin our lives because we have the choice to focus on what is good in each of us and to work positively, in attitude, with our genetic flaws. We can always choose to be a happy personality, who contributes to others to make the world a better place to live in. And we can experience life in ways other than what was preplanned before we got here. The fact is that we are where we are, because that is where we want to be, for the purpose of learning life lessons that will, hopefully, develop our soul.

When I am with a client, I do not lie down, nor do I go into trance. I am always in a state of heightened awareness, a part of the greater whole. It is very natural for me to tune into the collective unconscious, as Carl Jung called it, or to connect with Source, as Edgar Cayce did. While we are here on earth, a part of us is always in the spirit world, in the form of the Higher Self, or the Over Soul, which is our spiritual essence. When I dream, I am fully aware that I have been working at night in the spirit world and know exactly what I have been doing there. When I am awake, I can retrieve all the answers whenever I want them, through my soul's access to the universal askashic records which contain every thought, fact, act and utterance ever made.

If someone phones me with a question or writes to me for advice about a problem, I am able to assist them as well as if they had come to me in person. Although I have never worked with the police, I have been able to accurately answer questions for clients about missing people. When I am asked a question about a third party, I will give the answers about that person, if I think it is appropriate and not just a curiosity or an invasion of privacy and well-being.

Recently I had a phone call from a distraught woman concerning her sister who had a ferocious headache and was throwing up. She wanted to know if her sister had a brain aneurysm or internal hemorrhage. When I am called upon to help a sick person, I don't stop to think about whether the impressions I am getting are correct. My response is immediate and always accurate. I instantly knew that her sister had a violent migraine attack. I recommended that she handle the problem by putting rosemary and lavender oil on her sister's temples, a cold wet cloth on the back of her sister's neck and forehead, and to ask her sister to lie down in a dark room. Then I did a long distance healing on her sister. The next day, the woman called me back and said that she had followed my instructions, and her sister's migraine and vomiting had stopped at once. By the time the doctor had arrived, her sister was better, which is what I knew would happen.

Psychics and healers have various styles in the way they work. My friend, Maura Lundberg, a spiritual advisor and psychic, has x-ray vision like Cayce. She can actually see into the body to find out its condition. I cannot do that, but I can intuitively pick up on a person's aches, pains, disease, emotions and feelings, and without conscious thought processing will automatically suggest how to rectify whatever the problems are on a physical, mental, emotional or spiritual level. When I am concentrating on a healing, I do not give a psychic reading. But, whatever psychic information I pick up on that is relevant to the healing problem, I relate to the client.

You asked if I am able to access spirit beings? Well, Bette, there is a notion that psychics can call up the spirits of whomever they choose, but actually it doesn't work that way. Most of the time spirits appear to us when they choose to. But we can tune into our own Spirit Guides whenever we wish, or call upon our healing team of spiritual beings whenever we seek their help. I often call upon Mr. Cayce for help with clients or for myself, and he comes with the most obvious of answers. As for channeling between the two worlds, yes, I can do this, if the spirit involved wants to say something to the client, and if I think it is relevant to the person concerned. Psychics have to be very choosy about what they hear and pass on because some of the material that comes through is really of no importance to the person or situation under examination.

Shortly after Christmas this year I had a very strange and wonderful experience. While I was in bed, I saw a lady standing over me in midair. She seemed to get as much of a shock as I did. She said she didn't mean to scare me, and informed me that every night while I was asleep she was accustomed to working with me and a spiritual team of helpers. I already knew about this because I don't dream like others do. When I awaken in the morning, I can recall another world in which I work in at night.

The lady wanted to know if I was afraid. When I said no, she asked if she could bring in the others. "Please do!" I told her. The others then appeared around my bed. I realized that I was not dreaming, but actually in the presence of spiritual beings. While we are all spiritual beings, some of us have chosen to come to earth, and others choose to stay in the spirit world. Human beings and spiritual beings are all connected and can be of assistance to each other at all times.

When we come to earth, we are never left to drift alone. We always have a support system of guardian angels or a team of spiritual guides. They never interfere, dictate or try to control us. Their job is to try to guide us along our chosen path, whether we are aware of them or not. These spiritual beings that visited me were my team of guides. They talked to me about my life, work, wishes and dreams. We also discussed my teaching, and I asked a million and one questions. They agreed that we can teach others to do what I do, but not in the same way, because each person is unique and has a method of their own for accomplishing things.

We talked about spirituality, life, earth, the spirit world, our connection with each other, what it is to be spirit and to be human, and how we can all connect with Source at will. And we talked about psychics throughout the ages, including Edgar Cayce. My spirit guides, showed me the simplest of methods to teach communication with your guides. They asked me to pass this knowledge on to my students. First, clear your mind of thought as in the meditation state of no-thing-ness. If you have a question in mind for your guides, think it, don't presume an answer and don't analyze your own question. Release your question, and clear your mind of thought again. With the help of your guides the answer to your question will come from within you. When it does, don't analyze it, just accept it.

Ever since my night time discussion with my guides, I have been teaching students this language of communication with spirit guides and with themselves. Every person I have taught it to can do it perfectly.

I hope this gives you some idea of who Catherine Campbell, the psychic, healer, medium is, Bette.

May your life be blessed with love and light,

Catherine Campbell

....

Contact Catherine Campbell
about her spiritual mentoring,
psychism and healing classes, at:

catherinecampbell@eircom.net

....

Note by Catherine Campbell:

Years ago, before I began to help others as a psychic, healer and medium, I received a phone call from the author of *The Grand Design*, psychic Paddy McMahon, a man I had never heard of. He advised me that he could "see" my special God-given gifts, and that I was meant to use them in this lifetime to help people. He told me things about my life that nobody, other than myself, my Spirit Guide, or a gifted psychic like Paddy McMahon, could know. His friendship and encouragement have helped me live out my "grand design".

RECOMMENDED READING

Books by Paddy McMahon:

THE GRAND DESIGN
Vol. 1 (1987) and Vol. 2 (1991)
Hampton Roads

This series of books covers all aspects of our reason for being here and discusses spirit communication, afterlife, reincarnation and free will.

A FREE SPIRIT
Auricle Enterprises, 1999

This book was written with a spirit being known as Margaret Cussack. Her job is to welcome people into the spirit world when they move on.

Guidelines For Evaluating Psychic Information From The A.R.E.

Before a reading from a psychic, numerologist, astrologer, "guide", or from one's own dreams, inner guidance, visions, or intuition, formulate your questions to elicit clear answers. Begin by querying yourself with the following questions:

A) Why do I want this reading? Edgar Cayce indicated that the following factors play an incisive role in the clarity and depth of a reading: motivation or ideal behind the request for the reading, the psychic's purpose or ideal for giving the reading, the values of those most directly concerned with the person requesting the reading, and the psychic giving the reading. If the reading is prompted by greed, curiosity or desire for power, the quality, clarity and wisdom of the reading will be considerably less.

B) Am I looking for help to make my decisions or am I consciously or unconsciously trying to shift the responsibility to someone I think may be wiser and with a better view into my future? Getting someone else's perspective is often helpful when used for making informed decisions. A question to ask about your soul's purpose at a psychic reading is: What is my soul's purpose for this incarnation?

A question to ask about your past lifetimes at a psychic reading is: In order to fulfill my soul's purpose, please describe what past-life experiences and relationships I have had that most directly influence me in my current life and relationships?

Questions to ask at a psychic reading, about understanding specific interpersonal relationships or particular issues concerning a certain relationship, are: In order to attain real forgiveness and peace, how can I utilize past-life experiences constructively with (name the person you are referring to and include that person's birth date, birth time and birth place)? Or: What information can you give me that will help me understand the source of the problem that I am having with (name the person you are referring to and include that person's birth date, birth time and birth place), and how can I deal with the problem in order to experience love and healing in our relationship? Or: What are the prospects of being able to work well with (name the person you are referring to and include that person's birth date, birth time and birth place), and what potential pitfalls do you foresee in our relationship? Or: How can I understand and best relate to (name the person you are referring to and include that person's birth date, birth, time and birth place)?

Questions to ask about health concerns at a psychic reading: (**Note: Not every psychic is able to answer health questions. Even if the psychic can, it is best to use common sense in interpreting psychic guidance on health issues, and to also get advice from other medical sources.)** What areas of weakness, imbalance or illness in my body can you describe? And for each one, please tell me what I can do to promote healing in the ailing areas? Or: What is the cause, physically, mentally and spiritually, of my (name the disorder) problem? Or: What can I do to heal and balance my overall health?

Questions to ask at a psychic reading about transforming a particular attitude or emotion: Why do I lose my temper and how I can I learn to control it? Or: Why am I troubled with anxiety and insomnia? And what can I do about it?

Questions to ask at a psychic reading about the future: My ideal is (state what your ideal is). With that in mind, is my current place of employment the place that I can fulfill my work life ideal, or should I seek employment elsewhere? Or: My husband and I are considering having another child; should we? If so, how will our new child affect our current family? And will our child be a boy or a girl?

RECOGNIZING YOUR PSYCHIC DREAMS

1. Look for a symbol in your dream representing psychic or spiritual elements, like a crystal ball, a church or temple or a spiritually developed person.

2. The action in your dream may be symbolic and need interpretation. But the person you see in your dream may be the literal one you are trying to work out a problem with in your every day life.

3. Try to find the "red flags" in your dreams that mean ESP. For example, you may find that your dreams in vivid color have an ESP component, or that every time you dream about an airplane it is an ESP dream. Each person's clues are somewhat different. Only by studying your dreams will you discover the meaning of them.

4. Search your dreams for a psychic diagnosis of your physical health. Look for a part of the anatomy that you are dreaming about because it may be symbolic of a health diagnosis. Psychic dreams about health often manifest a hospital, clinic, doctor's office, bathroom (cleansing), kitchen or dining room (diet).

5. Look for a clock or other timepiece in your dream because they are signs about the future or distant past.

6. Seek past-life clues that come in vivid detail with costumes and settings from a different time and place, or more subtle clues like shoes or architecture from a different culture in another lifetime.

7. Look for the presence of a light, the symbol of dream contact with the superconscious mind or the God within. Other representations of this are: a wise old woman, Jesus, a mysterious bright light in the distance, the sun or other forms of light.

8. Examine your recurrent dreams. Although not every recurrent dream is literally predictive of a future event, the Cayce readings suggest that if we dream of something three or more times, we may expect it to be psychic in nature.

HOW TO EVALUATE PSYCHIC INFORMATION

Ask yourself the following questions:

1. Does the reading "ring true" for me? Did the psychic talk about confirmable facts?

2. Did the reading give me applicable things to try to do? If so, what are the results of trying them? Am I and other people involved benefited by these things?

3. Did the reading "call" me to be the best I know how to be in whatever I am doing in my life?

4. Did the reading empower me to take charge of my life, giving me a path to follow, rather than becoming dependent on the psychic?

5. Did the reading leave me with a sense of hope about my life, stretching me to new, unconsidered aspects of myself and my life?

6. Did the psychic information address me personally, using vocabulary, images and examples that I can relate to?

7. Allow someone who is a trusted friend to evaluate your questions to the psychic and the answers you received from the psychic. What is your friend's opinion of the questions and answers?

8. Did the psychic reading answer unasked questions that were within you?

9. Does the reading seem to get better with time?

RECOMMENDED READING

PARADOX OF POWER
Mark Thurston
(Helps answer the questions: What is my ideal?
and What is my soul's purpose?)
A.R.E. Press, 1987

THE EDGAR CAYCE IDEALS WORKBOOK
Kevin J. Todeschi
(Includes exercises and revealing self-quizzes
to help you in all aspects of daily living.)
A.R.E. Press, 1991

EDGAR CAYCE'S ESP
Kevin J. Todeschi, MA
and the Editors of the A.R.E.
A.R.E. Press, 1996

Index

Publisher's Related Books

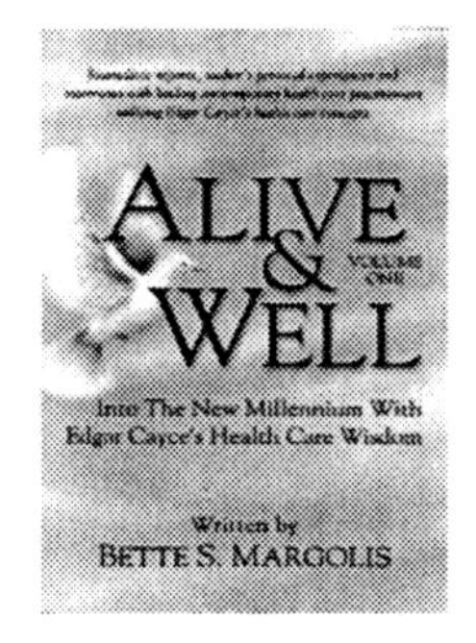

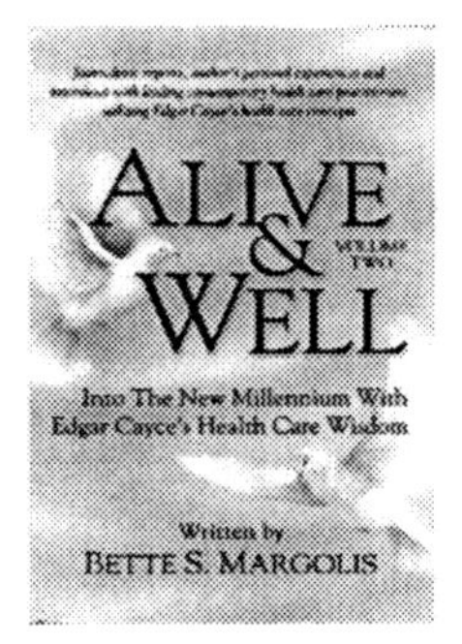

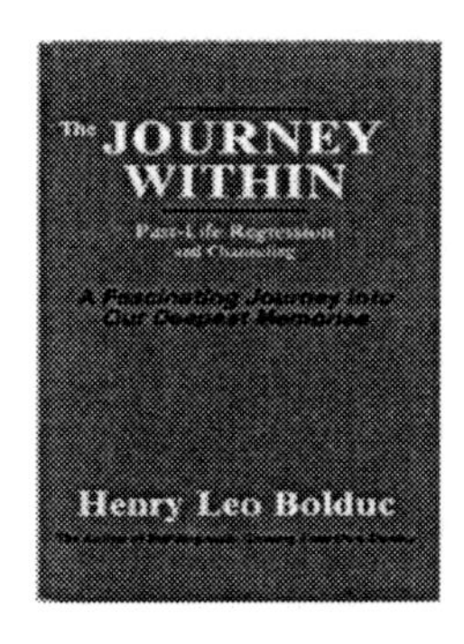

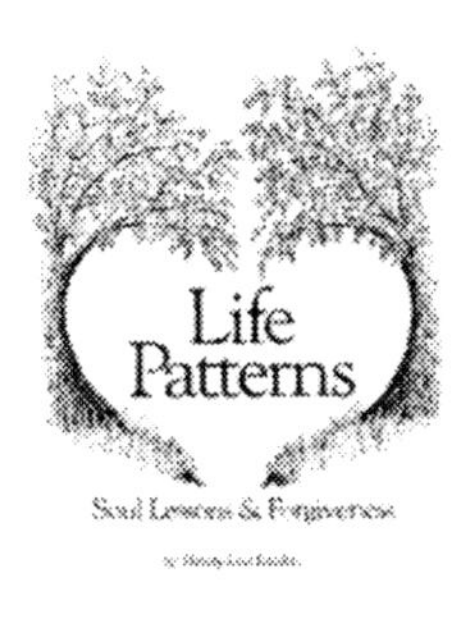

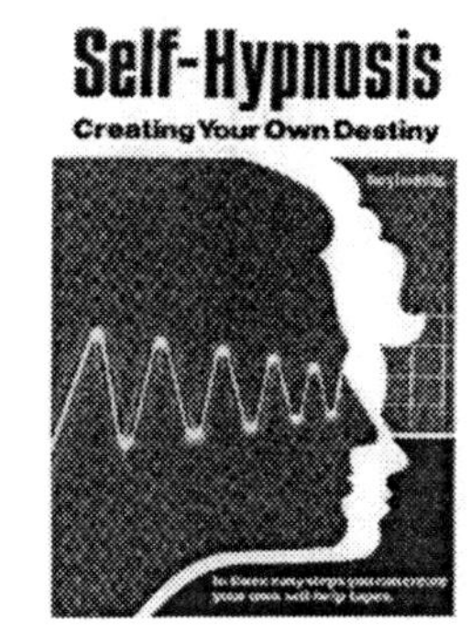

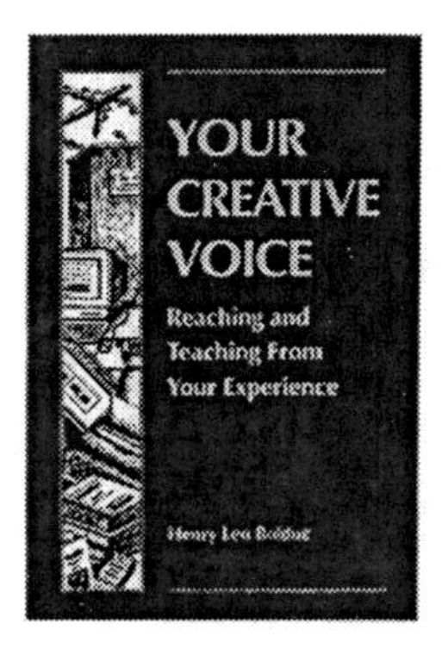

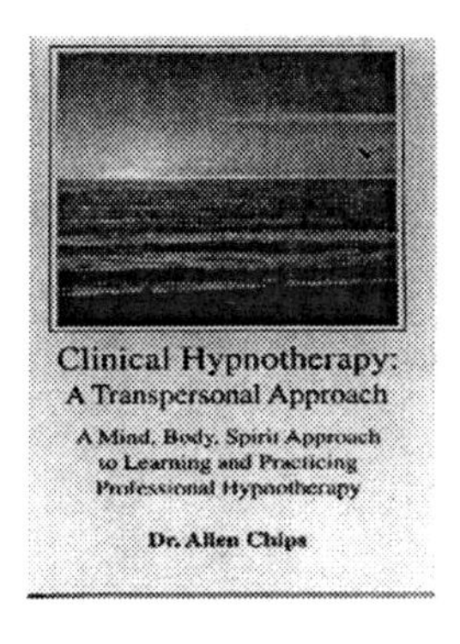

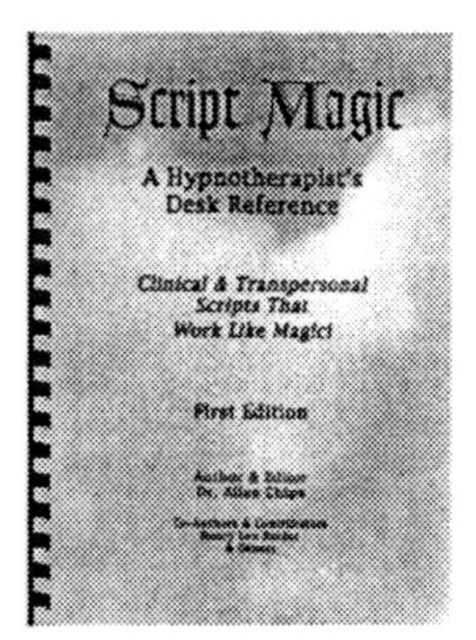

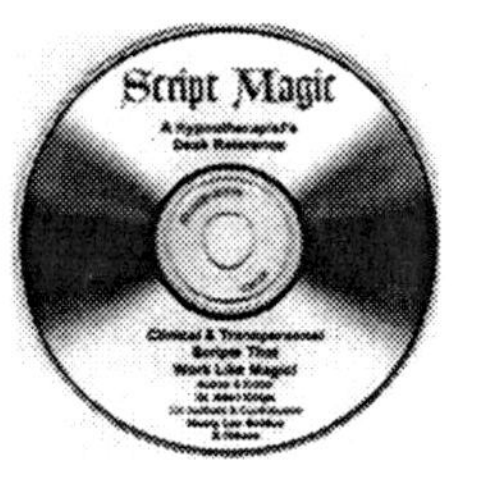

To direct order or contact the publisher
www.TranspersonalPublishing.com

Printed in the United States
93657LV00002B/400-417/A

9 781929 661138